Nutrition and Mental Health
A Complete Guide

Author Mary June Smith

Copyright © 2019 by Mary June Smith All Rights Reserved.

No part of this publication may be reproduced, distributed, or transmitted in any form or by any means, including photocopying, recording, or other electronic or mechanical methods, or by any information storage and retrieval system without the prior written permission of Smith Show Publishing, except in the case of very brief quotations embodied in critical reviews and certain other noncommercial uses permitted by copyright law.

Table of Contents

Regular Diet	5-7
Mechanical Soft (Dental Diet)	8-10
Dysphagia Level 1 (Pureed Diet	11-14
Dysphagia Level 2 (Mechanically Altered Diet)	15-19
Dysphagia Advanced Level 3 Diet	20-23
Full Liquid Diet	24-26
Clear Liquid Diet	27-28
Restricted Fiber Diet / Restricted Residue Diet	29-30
Increased Fiber Diet	31-33
Pleasure Feedings	34
Small Regular and Large Portion Sizes	35
Small Portions Diet	36-37
Large Portion Diet	38
Vegetarian Diet	39-41
Lacto-Ovovegetarian Meal Plan	42
Vegan Meal Plan	43
No Added Salt Diet	44
Low Sodium Diet (2 – 4 grams)	45
Cholesterol Restricted and Fat Controlled Diet	46-49
Limited K+ Diet & Liberalized Renal Diet	50
Renal Diet	51-53
Potassium Containing Foods (over 300 mg K+ per serving)	54-63
Renal Diet High Phosphorus Foods	64
Renal Diet Continued	65
Simplified Guideline for Standard Carbohydrate Controlled Diet	66-67
Carbohydrate Controlled Diet	68-95
Calorie Restricted (Low Calorie) Diet	96
Limited Concentrated Sweets (LCS) Diet	97-99
Diabetic Diet Calculated	100
Lactose Reduced Diet	101-102
Kosher Diet	103-107
Enteral Nutrition	108-110
Parenteral Nutrition	111-113
Gluten Free Diet	114-118
Finger Food Diet	119-122
Thickened Liquids	123

Appendix

Estimated Calorie Needs Method I	124-125
Estimated Calorie Needs Method II	126
Estimated Protein Needs	127-128
Miffin – St. Jeor Equation and Cheat Sheet	129
Estimated Fluid Needs/Serum Osmolality	130-131
Estimated Height	132
Nutrition Assessment Guidelines: When adjustments are required	133
Calculation Metabolically Active Weight and Ireton Jones Equation	134-135
References and Recommended Readings for Calculating Energy Needs	136
Body Mass Index & Table	137
MAO Inhibitors and Food Interactions	138-139
Fiber Content of Common Food	140-144
Recipes for Fiber Supplements	145
Caffeine Content of Foods and Beverages	146-147
Scoop Sizes	148
Milligrams and Milliequivalent Conversions	149
Measures and Metric Conversions	150
Abbreviations	151
Official "Do No Use" List	152-153
Recipe for Puree Bread	154-158
French Toast Souffle Recipe	159
Super Shake Recipe	160
Food Guide Pyramid, Dietary Guidelines for Americans 2005 and DASH Diet, DRI's 2010, My Plate For Older Adults, Information regarding risks of tube feeding for older adults and Culture Change Movement.	161

I. **Description**
The regular diet is designed for residents who do not require any dietary restrictions. The "Dietary Guidelines for Americans", 2010 and "My Plate for Older Adults" 2011 (see appendix) have been used as the basis for this and all other diets and menus in this edition. The meal patterns and daily amounts of each food group in the regular diet have been calculated to meet the needs of sedentary males and females age 51 and over. Refer to Appendix 5, 6, and 7 of the Dietary Guidelines for Americans 2010 to adjust the meal patterns for other age/gender and activity levels. Individual meal preferences must also be considered in planning this and other diets in the manual.

II. **Approximate Composition**
   Calories   1600-2000
   Protein   60-75 grams

III. **Adequacy**
This diet contains all nutrients necessary to provide and maintain adequate nutrition based on the Dietary Reference Intakes, 2010

FOOD GROUPS	FOODS INCLUDED	DAILY AMOUNTS
Milk	All types; yogurt	3 or more servings (1 serving equals 8 ounces)
Meat and equivalents	Meat, fish, shellfish, poultry, cheese, eggs, dried beans, peas and lentils, peanut butter, seeds, and nuts	At least 5 meat equivalents
		1 meat equivalent equals:
	Lean meats, fish, poultry no skin, lower fat cheeses	1 oz. cooked meat, fish, shellfish, ¼ cup canned tuna or salmon, 1 oz. poultry, 1 oz. cheese ¼ cup cottage or ricotta cheese, 1 egg, 2 egg whites
	Legumes and meat alternatives	½ cup cooked dried beans, peas, lentils, 2 tbsp peanut butter, 4 oz. of tofu;

Regular Diet

FOOD GROUPS	FOODS INCLUDED	DAILY AMOUNTS
Fruits	All types Citrus or high vitamin C fruit daily	2 or more servings 1 serving equals: ½ cup fruit, 1 medium fresh fruit or 4 ounces fruit juice
Vegetables	All types, including potatoes, corn, lima beans, peas; legumes, dark green leafy or yellow vegetables (3-4 times a week)	3 or more servings 1 serving equals: 1 cup chopped raw; or ½ cup cooked; or 4–6 ounces vegetable juice
Soups	All types	As desired 1 serving equals: 6 ounces
Bread, Cereal & Grains	All types, especially whole grains	6 or more servings 1 serving equals: 1 slice of bread; 3/4 cup ready to eat cereal; ½ cup cooked cereal; ½ cup rice, or ½ cup pasta
Fats	Oils, soft margarine, butter, (avoid trans-fat)	As needed for adequate caloric intake
Desserts	All types	As desired for adequate caloric intake
Beverages	All types, include 8 or more cups of water or other fluids per day	As needed to meet fluid requirement
Miscellaneous	Sugar, condiments, jam, jelly, preserves, syrup, sweets, herbs, spices, flavorings, salt, pepper	As desired for flavor and palatability

Regular Diet

Sample Menu Plan
Breakfast

Fruit or juice	Orange juice	4 ounces
Cereal	Oatmeal	½ cup
Meat or equivalent	Eggs, scrambled	1
Bread	Toast, whole wheat	1 slice
Fat	Soft margarine	1 packet
Milk	Milk, 2%	8 ounces
Beverage	Beverage of choice	6-8 ounces
Miscellaneous	Jelly	1 tablespoon
	Sugar	2 packets
	Creamer	as desired
	Salt, Pepper	1 packet each

Lunch or Supper

Meat or Equivalent	Tuna salad	½ cup
Vegetable	Vegetable soup	6 ounces
Salad	Tossed salad	1 cup
Fat	Italian dressing	1 ounce
Bread	Whole wheat bread	2 slices
Dessert	Chilled peaches	½ cup
Milk	Milk, 2%	8 ounces
Miscellaneous	Beverage of choice	6-8 ounces
	Sugar	1-2 packets
	Creamer	as desired
	Salt, Pepper	1 packet each

Dinner

Meat or equivalent	Baked chicken breast	½ breast (3 ounces)
Potato	Mashed potatoes, gravy	½ cup, 1 ounce
Vegetable	Seasoned carrots	½ cup
Salad	Mixed fruit salad	½ cup
Bread	Dinner roll, whole wheat	1
Fat	Soft margarine	1 packet
Milk	Milk, 2%	8 ounces
Dessert	Vanilla ice cream	½ cup
Beverage	Beverage of choice	6-8 ounces
Miscellaneous	Sugar	1-2 packets
	Creamer	as desired
	Salt, Pepper	1 packet each

Evening Nourishment

	Juice	4 ounces
	Graham crackers	3 squares

I. Description
This diet modifies the consistency of the regular diet and is used when an individual has difficulty chewing regular food. Most foods on the regular diet may be included, with mechanical alterations based on individual tolerance.

II. Approximate Composition
Calories   1600-2000
Protein   60-75 grams

III. Adequacy
This diet provides all nutrients necessary based on the Dietary Guidelines for Americans 2010.

FOOD GROUPS	FOODS INCLUDED	FOODS EXCLUDED
Milk	All types; yogurt	None
Meat and Equivalent	Ground meat & poultry (gravy/sauces may be added to moisten); soft boneless fish; ground meat casseroles; cheese sauce, soft cheese, cottage cheese; shaved luncheon meat; eggs; creamy peanut butter; meat loaf/ham loaf, Salisbury Steak; finely chopped meat, tuna or egg salads	Whole meats, whole hot dogs, hard cheeses; any other difficult-to-chew foods
Fruit	All fruit juices, cooked or canned fruit, soft fresh fruit as tolerated	Dried fruits; hard fresh fruits
Vegetables	All vegetable juices; well-cooked soft vegetables: chopped or diced; shredded salads as tolerated	Whole raw vegetables; corn on the cob
Soups	All types	Any not tolerated
Bread & Cereal & Grains	Breads, crackers, dry cereals; French toast, pancakes and waffles with syrup; doughnuts, muffins without nuts/seeds, croissants, pastries without nuts or dried fruit	Granola or granola-type cereals, any foods with nuts or dried fruits, bagels

Mechanical Soft (Dental) Diet

FOOD GROUPS	FOODS INCLUDED	FOODS EXCLUDED
Potatoes & Starches	Baked, boiled or mashed potatoes, french fries; pasta	Wild rice
Fats	All types, crisp bacon as tolerated	None
Desserts	Most types	Any containing nuts, coconut, or dried fruit
Beverages	All types	None
Miscellaneous	Herbs, spices, salt, pepper gravies/sauces, ketchup, mayonnaise, mustard, pickle slices	Nuts, coconut, whole pickles, popcorn

Sample Menu Plan

Breakfast

Fruit or juice	Orange juice	4 ounces
Cereal	Oatmeal	½ cup
Meat or equivalent	Egg, scrambled	1
Bread	Whole wheat toast	1 slice
Fat	Soft margarine	1 packet
Milk	Milk, 2%	8 ounces
Beverage	of choice	6-8 ounces
Miscellaneous	Jelly	1 tablespoon
	Sugar	2 packets
	Creamer	as desired
	Salt, Pepper	1 packet each

Lunch or Supper

Meat or equivalent	Finely chopped tuna salad	½ cup
Vegetable	Vegetable soup	6 ounces
Salad	Shredded tossed salad	½ cup
Potato or equivalent	Sweet potatoes	½ cup
Fat	Italian dressing	1 ounce
Bread	Whole wheat bread	2 slices
Dessert	Chilled peaches	½ cup
Milk	Milk, 2%	8 ounces
Beverage	of choice	6-8 ounces
Miscellaneous	Sugar	1-2 packets
	Creamer	as desired
	Salt, Pepper	1 packet each

Dinner

Meat or equivalent	Moist ground chicken breast with gravy	3 ounces / 1 ounce
Potato or Equivalent	Mashed potatoes/gravy	½ cup/1 ounce
Vegetable	Cooked sliced carrots	½ cup
Fruit	Canned fruit salad	½ cup
Bread	Soft dinner roll	1
Fat	Soft margarine	1 packet
Milk	Milk, 2%	8 ounces
Dessert	Vanilla ice cream	½ cup
Beverage	of choice	6-8 ounces
	Sugar	1-2 packets
	Creamer	as desired
	Salt, pepper	1 packet each

Evening Nourishment

	Apple juice	4 ounces
	Graham crackers	3 squares

I. **Description**
The pureed diet is used for individuals who have difficulty chewing and/or swallowing. Any foods from the regular diet that can be appropriately pureed should be included in this diet. Individuals requiring a pureed diet simply due to chewing difficulties may be able to tolerate additional food items on an individual basis. This should be specified in the individual's care plan. Procedures should be developed for pureeing food to provide correct and adequate portions equivalent to the portions used in a regular diet. The consistency should be smooth and thick enough to mound on the plate, and similar in consistency to that of pudding.
*NOTE: Additional modifications may be required if the individuals are on thickened liquids.

II. **Approximate Composition**
Calories   1600-2000
Protein   60-75 grams

III. **Adequacy**
This diet provides all nutrients necessary to provide and maintain adequate nutrients based on the Dietary Guidelines for Americans 2010.

FOOD GROUPS	FOODS INCLUDED	FOODS EXCLUDED
Milk	All types; yogurt without chunks, seeds or nuts	Any yogurt containing chunks of fruit, coconut, nuts or seeds
Meat and equivalents	Pureed meat, eggs, fish, and poultry; soufflés that are homogenous and smooth; hummus or other pureed legumes; softened tofu; Braunschweiger, pureed cheese and pureed cottage cheese; creamy peanut butter mixed with other pureed food; pureed eggs	Whole or ground meats, fish or poultry; non-pureed lentils or legumes; peanut butter (unless pureed into foods correctly); non-pureed fried, cooked or scrambled eggs
Fruits	Pureed fruits, fruit juices without pulp, well-mashed fresh bananas	Whole fruits (fresh, frozen, canned or dried); juices with pulp
Vegetables	Pureed vegetables, vegetable juices with pulp or seeds	All other non-pureed vegetables, including those with seeds or hulls that cannot be properly pureed
Soups	Broth, bouillon, Strained or pureed soups	Non-pureed soups with lumps or chunks

FOOD GROUPS	FOODS INCLUDED	FOODS EXCLUDED
Bread, Cereal, & Grains	Pureed bread mixes; pregelled slurried breads, pancakes, French toast, danish, pastries, sweet rolls, etc. that are softened throughout entire thickness of product.	All other breads, rolls crackers, pancakes, waffles, biscuits, muffins etc.
	Smooth, homogenous cooked cereals, such as farina-type cereals. Cereals should have a "pudding-like" consistency	All dry cereals and cooked cereals with chunks, lumps or seeds; oatmeal
Potatoes & Starches	Mashed potatoes; Pureed potatoes (moistened with gravy, butter, margarine or sour cream for individuals with dysphagia)	All others
	Pureed well-cooked pasta, Noodles, bread dressing or rice (blenderized to a smooth homogenous consistency.	
Fats	Butter, margarine, mayonnaise, cream cheese, whipped topping, strained gravy, sour cream	Any fats with course or chunky additives
	Smooth sauces, such as cheese sauce, white sauce, or hollandaise sauce	

FOOD GROUPS	FOODS INCLUDED	FOODS EXCLUDED
Desserts	Smooth custards, puddings and yogurt	Fruited yogurt, cookies, cakes, pies, pastries, course or textured puddings, bread puddings pies
	Pureed desserts and soufflés, fruit whips	
	* Ice cream sherbet, ices gelatins, milk shakes/malts, eggnog, frozen yogurt, and nutritional supplements * *Items that are liquid at room temperature may not be appropriate for individuals requiring thickened beverages*	
Beverages	Smooth, homogenous Beverages without lumps, Chunks or pulp.	All other beverages
Miscellaneous	Sugar, sugar substitute, salt, finely ground pepper and spices	Coarsely ground pepper and herbs
	Catsup, mustard, barbeque sauce and other smooth sauces and gravies	Seeds, nuts, sticky foods, sauces with lumps, etc.
	Clear jam, jelly, syrup, and honey	Chunky fruit preserves and jams/jellies with seeds
	Very soft, smooth candy	Candy with nuts, sprinkles, etc.; chewy candies such as caramels or licorice

* **Pureed bread recipes in appendix**
***Most beverages and soups will need to be thickened for individuals requiring thickened liquids. This includes all items that are liquid at room temperature, such as ice cream, shakes, gelatin, etc.**

Sample Menu Plan
Breakfast

Fruit or juice	Orange juice	4 ounces
Cereal	Cream of wheat	½ cup
Meat or equivalent	Pureed egg,	1
Bread	Slurried bread	1 slice
Fat	Margarine	1 teaspoon
Milk	Milk, 2%	8 ounces
Beverage	of choice	6-8 ounces
Miscellaneous	Sugar	2 packets
	Creamer	as desired
	Salt, Pepper	1 packet each

Lunch and Supper

Meat or Equivalent	Pureed tuna salad	½ cup
Vegetable	Pureed vegetable soup	6 ounces
	Pureed beets	½ cup
Bread	Pureed bread	1 slice
Fat	Margarine	1 teaspoon
Dessert	Pureed Peaches	½ cup
Beverage	of choice	6-8 ounces
Milk	Milk, 2%	8 ounces
Miscellaneous	Sugar	1-2 packets
	Creamer	as desired
	Salt, Pepper	1 packet each

Dinner

Meat or equivalent	Pureed skinless baked chicken	½ cup (3 ounces edible)*
	Gravy	1 ounce
Potato or equivalent	Whipped potatoes w/ gravy	½ cup
Vegetable	Pureed carrots	½ cup
Bread	Pureed bread	1 serving
Fat	Margarine	1 teaspoon
Milk	Milk, 2%	8 ounces
Dessert	Vanilla ice cream	½ cup
Beverage	of choice	6-8 ounces
	Sugar	1-2 packet
	Creamer	as desired
	Salt, Pepper	1 packet each

Evening Nourishment

	Vanilla pudding	½ cup
	Apple juice	½ cup

*Portion size is based on a standardized procedure for pureeing cooked chicken to provide 3 meat equivalents.

I. **Description**
This diet consists of foods that are moist and easily formed into a bolus. Meats (ground or minced) should be no larger than one-quarter inch pieces. All foods from the Dysphagia Level 1/pureed diet are acceptable on this diet. It is based on the National Dysphagia Diet Level 2 Dysphagia Mechanically Altered diet, and is designed for individuals who have difficulty swallowing regular foods. It is designed to be a transition from pureed to more solid textures. Some mixed textures are acceptable on this diet, and chewing ability is required. Individuals should be monitored periodically to determine if swallowing function improves or declines.
*NOTE: Additional modifications may be required if the individuals are on thickened liquids.

II. **Approximate Composition**
Calories   1600-2000
Protein   60-75 grams

III. **Adequacy**
This diet provides all nutrients necessary based on the Dietary Guidelines for Americans 2010.

FOOD GROUPS	FOODS INCLUDED	FOODS EXCLUDED
Milk	All types – Beverages may require thickening when thin liquids are to be avoided	None
Meat and Equivalent	Moist ground meats or poultry; moist soft fish; casseroles without rice; moist macaroni and cheese; well-cooked pasta with meat sauce; soft moist lasagna; moist meatballs, meat loaf, ham or fish loaf; protein salads without large chunks, celery, or onion; cottage cheese; smooth quiche without large chunks; scrambled eggs; poached pasteurized eggs; soft soufflés; tofu; well-cooked slightly mashed moist legumes, such as baked beans; All meat or protein substitutes should be served with sauces or moistened.	Dry or tough meats such as bacon, hot dogs, sausage, and bratwurst Dry casseroles, casseroles with rice or large chunks Cheese slices and cubes; hard-cooked or crisp fried eggs; Sandwiches; pizza Peanut butter

FOOD GROUPS	FOODS INCLUDED	FOODS EXCLUDED
Fruit	Soft drained canned or cooked fruits without seeds or skin; soft/ripe banana; fruit juice	Fresh or frozen fruits, cooked fruits with skins or seeds; dried fruits; fresh, canned or cooked pineapple
Vegetable	Soft, well-cooked vegetables, less than ½ inch in size and should be easily mashed with a fork; vegetable juices	Cooked corn and peas; broccoli, cabbage, asparagus, Brussels sprouts, or other fibrous, nontender/rubbery raw or cooked vegetables
Soups	Soups with easy-to-chew/swallow meats or vegetables; particle size in soups should be less than ½ inch Soups may require thickening for residents on thickened liquids	Soups with large chunks of meat and vegetables; soups with rice, corn or peas
Bread, Cereal & Grains	Soft pancakes moistened with syrup or sauce; pureed bread mixes, pregelled or slurried breads that are gelled throughout entire thickness of product	All other breads
	Cooked cereals with little texture, including oatmeal; slightly moistened dry cereals with little texture, such as corn flakes, Rice Krispies ®, Wheaties®, etc.	Very course cooked cereals that contain nuts or seeds; whole-grain dry or coarse cereals; cereals with nuts, seeds, dried fruit and/or coconut
	Un-processed wheat bran stirred into cereals for bulk- Liquid should be absorbed into the product when thin liquids are contraindicated.	

FOOD GROUPS	FOODS INCLUDED	FOODS EXCLUDED
Potatoes and Starches	Well-cooked, moistened, Baked, boiled, or mashed potatoes	Potato skins and chips; fried or french-fried potatoes; rice
	Well-cooked noodles in sauce; soft dumplings moistened with butter, sauce or gravy; well-cooked shredded hash browns (not crisp) in sauce	
Fats	Butter, margarine, cream, Gravy, sauces, mayonnaise, salad dressing, sour cream, whipped toppings, cream cheese, dip and spreads with soft additives - Thickening agents may be required when thin liquids are contraindicated	Any fats with coarse, chunky additives
Desserts	Pudding, custard, soft fruit pies with bottom crust only; pre-gelled cookies, or soft cookies that have been moistened in milk, coffee, or other liquid; soft-moist cakes with icing, or slurried cakes; crisps and cobblers with soft breading or crumb mixture (without seeds or nuts); Frozen yogurt, ice cream, sherbets, ices, malts, milk shakes, eggnog, gelatin and nutritional supplements – items that are liquid at room temperature may require thickening when thin liquids are contraindicated	Pineapple; any foods with dried fruit, nuts, coconut, or seeds

FOOD GROUPS	FOODS INCLUDED	FOODS EXCLUDED
Beverages	All beverages with minimal amounts of texture, pulp, etc. Milk, juice, coffee, tea, soda, alcoholic beverages, nutritional supplements – liquids may require thickening if thin liquids are contraindicated	
Miscellaneous	Jams and preserves without seeds; jelly	Seeds, nuts, coconut, sticky foods
	Sauces, salsas, etc. that may have small tender chunks less than ½ inch in size	Chewy candies such as caramel or licorice
	Soft, smooth chocolate bars that are easily chewed	

Sample Menu Plan
Breakfast

Fruit or juice	Orange juice	4 ounces
Cereal	Oatmeal	½ cup
Meat or equivalent	Egg, scrambled	1
Bread	Pureed bread	1 serving
Fat	Soft margarine	1 packet
Milk	Milk, 2%	8 ounces
Beverage	of choice	6-8 ounces
Miscellaneous	Jelly	1 tablespoon
	Sugar	1-2 packets
	Creamer	as desired
	Salt, Pepper	1 packet each

Lunch or Supper

Meat or equivalent	Soft flaked fish with sauce	3 ounces/1 ounce
Vegetable	Green beans	½ cup
Potato or equivalent	Mashed potatoes/gravy	½ cup/1 ounce
Bread	Pureed bread	1 serving
Fruit	Canned peaches	½ cup
Fat	Soft margarine	1 packet
Milk	Milk, 2%	8 ounces
Beverage	of choice	6-8 ounces
Miscellaneous	Sugar	1-2 packets
	Creamer	as desired
	Salt, Pepper	1 packet each

Dinner

Meat or equivalent	Moist ground chicken/gravy	3 ounces/1 ounce
Potato or equivalent	Whipped potatoes/gravy	½ cup/1 ounce
Vegetable	Cooked sliced carrots	½ cup
Fruit	Canned fruit without pineapple	½ cup
Bread	Puree bread	1 serving
Fat	Soft margarine	1 packet
Milk	Milk, 2%	8 ounces
Dessert	Vanilla ice cream	½ cup
Beverage	of choice	6-8 ounces
Miscellaneous	Sugar	1-2 packets
	Creamer	as desired
	Salt, Pepper	1 packet each

Evening Nourishment

	Vanilla pudding	½ cup
	Apple juice	½ cup

I. **Description**
This diet consists of food of nearly regular textures with the exception of very hard, sticky or crunchy foods. Foods should be moist and in "bite-size" pieces. It is meant to be a transition to a regular diet. Adequate dentition and mastication are required. It is expected that mixed textures are tolerated on this diet. This diet is based on the National Dysphagia Diet Level 3 Dysphagia Advanced diet.

*NOTE: Additional modifications may be required if the individuals are on thickened liquids.

II. **Approximate Composition**
Calories   1600-2000
Protein   60-75 grams

III. **Adequacy**
This diet provides all nutrients necessary based on the Dietary Guidelines for Americans 2010.

FOOD GROUPS	FOODS INCLUDED	FOODS EXCLUDED
Milk	All types – Beverages may require thickening when thin liquids are contraindicated	None
Meat and Equivalent	Thin-sliced, tender or ground meats and poultry	Tough, dry meats and poultry
	Well-moistened fish	Dry fish, fish w/ bones
	Eggs prepared any way	Chunky peanut butter
	Yogurt without nuts/coconut	Yogurt w/ nuts or coconut
	Casseroles with small chunks of meat, ground meats or tender meats	

FOOD GROUPS	FOODS INCLUDED	FOODS EXCLUDED
Fruit	All canned and cooked fruits	Difficult to chew fruits, e.g. apples or pears
	Soft, peeled fresh fruits, e.g. peaches, kiwi, melons without seeds, nectarines	Stringy, high-pulp fruits, e.g. papaya, pineapple, mango
	Soft berries w/ small seeds such as strawberries	Fresh fruits w/ difficult to chew skins, such as grapes
		Uncooked dried fruits, e.g. prunes, apricots
		Fruit leather, fruit roll-ups, fruits snacks, dried fruits
Vegetable	All cooked, tender vegetables	Raw vegetables except shredded lettuce
	Shredded lettuce	Cooked corn
		Nontender or rubbery cooked vegetables
Soups	All soups except those on the excluded list	Soups w/ tough meats
		Corn or clam chowders
	Strained corn or clam chowder (may require thickening if thin liquids are contraindicated)	Soups w/ large chunks of meat or vegetables > 1 inch
Bread, Cereal & Grains	Well-moistened breads, biscuits, muffins, pancakes, Waffles, etc. Need to add Adequate syrup, butter, jelly, etc. to moisten sufficiently	Dry bread, toast, crackers, etc.
		Tough, crusty breads, e.g. French bread or baguettes
	All well-moistened cereals (May have ¼ cup milk or just enough to moisten if thin liquids are restricted)	Course or dry cereals, e.g. Shredded Wheat or All Bran

FOOD GROUPS	FOODS INCLUDED	FOODS EXCLUDED
Potatoes & Starches	All – including rice, wild rice moist bread dressing, tender, fried potatoes	Tough, crisp-fried potatoes Potato skins Dry bread dressing
Fats	All fats except those on the excluded list	Fats w/ course, difficult-to-chew or chunky additives, e.g. cream cheese spread with nuts or pineapple
Desserts	All desserts except those on the excluded list *Malts, milk shakes, frozen yogurt, ice cream, gelatin, nutritional supplements, sherbet *These items become thin liquids at room and/or body temperature, and should be avoided if thin liquids are contraindicated	Dry cakes, cookies that are chewy or very dry Anything w/ nuts, seeds, dry Fruits, coconut, pineapple
Beverages	Any – depending on Recommendations for liquid consistency	
Miscellaneous	All seasonings & sweeteners All sauces Non-chewy candies without nuts, seeds, or coconut Jams, jellies, honey, preserves	Nuts, seeds, coconut Chewy, caramel or taffy-type candies Candies w/ nuts, seeds or coconut

Sample Menu Plan

Breakfast

Fruit or juice	Orange juice	4 ounces
Cereal	Oatmeal	½ cup
Meat or equivalent	Egg, scrambled	1
Bread	Whole wheat toast	1 slice
Fat	Soft margarine	1 packet
Milk	Milk, 2%	8 ounces
Beverage	of choice	6-8 ounces
Miscellaneous	Jelly	1 tablespoon
	Sugar	1-2 packets
	Creamer	as desired
	Salt, Pepper	1 packet each

Lunch or Supper

Meat or equivalent	Soft flaked fish with sauce	3 ounces/1 ounce
Vegetable	Green beans	½ cup
Potato or equivalent	Mashed potatoes/gravy	½ cup/1 ounce
Bread	whole wheat bread	1 slice
Fruit	Canned peaches	½ cup
Fat	Soft margarine	1 packet
Milk	Milk, 2%	8 ounces
Beverage	of choice	6-8 ounces
Miscellaneous	Sugar	1-2 packets
	Creamer	as desired
	Salt, Pepper	1 packet each

Dinner

Meat or equivalent	Tender chicken/gravy	3 ounces/1 ounce
Potato or equivalent	Whipped potatoes/gravy	½ cup/1 ounce
Vegetable	Cooked sliced carrots	½ cup
Fruit	Canned fruit without pineapple	½ cup
Bread	Dinner roll, whole wheat	1 serving
Fat	Soft margarine	1 packet
Milk	Milk, 2%	8 ounces
Dessert	Vanilla ice cream	½ cup
Beverage	of choice	6-8 ounces
Miscellaneous	Sugar	1-2 packets
	Creamer	as desired
	Salt, Pepper	1 packet each

Evening Nourishment

	Vanilla pudding	½ cup
	Apple juice	½ cup

I. **Description**
The full liquid diet consists of foods that are primarily liquid. This diet is indicated for residents who are acutely ill or who are unable to swallow or chew solid foods. Nourishments are served between meals. After 3-5 days, the need for this diet should be evaluated to assure adequate nutrition. If circumstances indicate that this diet is required for any extended period of time commercially prepared, nutritionally adequate supplements should become an essential component of this diet.

II. **Approximate Composition**
Calories   Varies
Protein   Varies

III. **Adequacy**
This diet may not contain all nutrients necessary to provide and maintain adequate nutrition based on the Dietary Guidelines for Americans 2010.

FOOD GROUPS	FOODS INCLUDED	FOODS EXCLUDED
Milk	All types; cocoa, hot chocolate, milk shakes, instant breakfast, eggnog, smooth yogurt (plain or flavored	Yogurt, with nuts, seeds, skins, whole fruits
Meat and Equivalents	Eggs or egg substitutes in custard or pudding	All others
Fruits	All juices and nectars without pulp	All others
Vegetables	Vegetable juices, vegetable purees that are strained in soups	All others

Full Liquid Diet

FOOD GROUPS	FOODS INCLUDED	FOODS EXCLUDED
Soups	Bouillon, broth; strained meat, vegetable and cream soups	All others
Cereals	Cooked refined cereals; strained oatmeal thinned with liquid	All others
Fats	Margarine or butter, cream, or non-dairy creamer	All others
Desserts	Pudding, custard, gelatin; plain ice cream, ice milk, sherbet, fruit ice; popsicles; plain frozen yogurt; commercially prepared pudding-type nutritional supplements	All others
Beverages	All types including commercially prepared liquid nutritional supplements	None
Miscellaneous	Sugar, clear jelly, syrup, honey; hard candy (if tolerated), chocolate syrup Salt, pepper	None

Sample Menu Plan

Breakfast

Fruit	Orange juice, pulp free	8 ounces
Cereal	Oatmeal	1 cup
Milk	Milk, 2%	8 ounces
Beverage	of choice	6-8 ounces
Miscellaneous	Sugar	3 packets
	Creamer	as desired

Midmorning Nourishment — Commercial liquid supplement — 8 ounces

Lunch & Supper

Fruit Juice	Apple juice	8 ounces
Soup	Strained vegetable soup	8 ounces
Dessert	lemon pudding	½ cup
Milk	Milk, 2%	8 ounces
Beverage	of choice	6-8 ounces
Miscellaneous	Sugar	3 packets
	Creamer	as desired
	Salt, pepper	1 packet each

Midmorning Nourishment — Commercial liquid supplement — 8 ounces

Dinner

Juice	Cranberry juice	8 ounces
Soup	Strained cream of mushroom soup	6 ounces
Dessert	vanilla ice cream	½ cup
Milk	Milk, 2%	8 ounces
Beverage	of choice	6-8 ounces
Miscellaneous	Sugar	2 packets
	Creamer	as desired
	Salt, pepper	1 packet each

Evening Nourishment

	Sherbet	½ cup
	Ginger ale	8 ounces

I. **Description**
The clear liquid diet is used for acute stages of illness until a full liquid diet or solid foods are tolerated. Nourishments between meals are necessary.

II. **Approximate Composition**
Calories   Varies
Protein   Varies

III. **Adequacy**
This diet is inadequate in all nutrients. It should be used for limited periods of time, usually no longer than 48 hours.

FOODS INCLUDED	FOODS EXCLUDED
Clear broth, bouillon	All others
Flavored gelatin	
High protein gelatin	
Water ice, popsicles, fruit ice	
Fruit juices: apple, grape, cranberry juice Cocktail, cran-apple, cran-grape, cran-raspberry, Orange or grapefruit juice without pulp	
Beverages: water, tea, coffee, carbonated beverages, fruit flavored drinks, commercially prepared high protein clear liquid products	
Sugar, sugar substitutes	

Sample Menu Plan
Breakfast

Pulp free orange juice	8 ounces
Cherry gelatin	1 cup
Carbonated cola	8 ounces
Beverage of choice	6-8 ounces
Ice water	8 ounces
Sugar	3 packets

Midmorning Nourishment

Grape juice	8 ounces
Raspberry gelatin	½ cup

Lunch

Apple juice	8 ounces
Chicken broth	6 ounces
Lemon ice	½ cup
Beverage of choice	6-8 ounces
Iced water	8 ounces
Sugar	3 packets

Mid Afternoon Nourishment

Pulp free orange juice	8 ounces
Lemon-lime	8 ounces
Carbonated beverage	

Dinner

Cranberry juice	8 ounces
Beef bouillon	6 ounces
Cherry gelatin	1 cup
Beverage of choice	6-8 ounces
Iced water	8 ounces
Sugar	3 packets

Evening Nourishment

Lime gelatin	1 cup
Ginger ale	8 ounces

I. **Description**

The fiber restricted diet limits the amount of dietary fiber. The purpose for using the fiber restricted diet is to decrease stool weight, fecal output and frequency. The restricted fiber diet may be used for the short-term treatment of acute ulcerative colitis, regional enteritis (Crohn's disease), acute diverticulitis and as necessary for bowel rest. This diet is used as a temporary measure during the transition to a regular diet. Once symptoms subside, high fiber foods should be gradually added to the diet. This diet should be tailored to the individual resident based on food preferences, tolerances and type of illness. The fiber restricted diet provides 15 grams or less of fiber per day. Milk, meat, fish, poultry, eggs and beverages provide little or no dietary fiber and can be included in this diet without restriction when planning the low fiber diet follow the guidelines for the regular diet for minimum daily amounts of these and other food groups. Substitute lower fiber content foods by following these guidelines:

1. Include only white or refined breads and cereals; omit all whole wheat and whole grain breads and cereals and products containing bran.

2. Include fruit and vegetable juices without pulp (omit prune juice), canned or cooked fruits; omit raw or dried fruit and all berries.

3. Include most well cooked vegetables without seeds (omit sauerkraut, winter squash, peas, corn and raw vegetables).

4. Omit dried beans and peas, lentils, legumes, peanut butter, and any foods containing seeds, nuts, coconut and dried fruits.

5. Limit milk to 2 cups/day.

II. **Approximate Composition**
Calories   1600-2000
Protein   60-75 grams
Fiber   15 grams or less

III. **Adequacy**
Depending on individual food choices and tolerances, the diet is adequate in all nutrients based on the Dietary Guidelines for Americans 2010. However, the Dietary Reference Intake (DRI) for iron will not be met for pregnant, lactating and pre-menopausal women following this diet. Residents on restricted fiber diets may need to be supplemented with ascorbic acid, folate and magnesium.

Restricted Fiber Diet

Sample Menu Plan
Breakfast

Fruit or Juice	Orange juice (pulp free)	4 ounces
Cereal	Corn flakes	1 cup
Meat or equivalent	Egg, scrambled	1
Bread	Toast, white	1 slice
Fat	Soft margarine	1 packet
Milk	Milk, 2%	8 ounces
Beverage	of choice	6-8 ounces
Miscellaneous	Jelly	1 tablespoon
	Sugar	2 packets
	Creamer	as desired
	Salt, Pepper	1 packet

Lunch

Soup	Cream of tomato soup	6 ounces
Meat or equivalent	Plain tuna salad with mayo.	½ cup
Bread	White bread	2 slices
Salad	Pickled beets, canned	½ cup
Fat	Soft margarine	1 packet
Dessert	Chilled peaches	½ cup
Beverage	Cold or Hot	8 ounces
Miscellaneous	Sugar, Salt, Pepper	1 packet each

Dinner

Meat or equivalent	Baked chicken breast	3 ounces
Vegetable	Carrots, cooked	½ cup
	Vegetable juice	½ cup
Starch	Mashed potatoes	½ cup
Bread	Roll/ white bread	1
Milk	Milk, 2%	8 ounces
Beverage	Cold or Hot	8 ounces
Dessert	Water ice	½ cup
Iced water		8 ounces
Miscellaneous	Sugar, Salt, Pepper	1 packet each

Evening Nourishment

	Juice	4 ounces
	Graham Crackers	3 squares

Increased Fiber Diet

I. **Description**

This diet emphasizes the use of high fiber food sources such as whole grain breads and cereals, fruits, vegetables, dried beans and peas. The purpose for using the increased fiber diet is to promote normal bowel function. Fiber adequately decreases the transit time of foods through the gastrointestinal tract and, with adequate fluid intake, results in soft stools. Dietary fiber is the portion of plant materials which is resistant to digestive enzymes in the body and includes cellulose, hemicellulose, lignin and pectin. The increased fiber diet may be used for the treatment of diverticulosis*, mild diverticulitis*, hemorrhoids, irritable bowel syndrome, diarrhea and constipation. When planning the increased fiber diet, follow the daily amounts of the food groups on the regular diet. Substitute higher fiber content foods by following these guidelines:

1. Include 1 serving of high fiber cereal (5 gms. of fiber or more) such as raisin bran, oatmeal, all bran, per day at breakfast or as a bedtime snack. Top with fruit for more fiber.

2. Choose whole wheat or whole grain breads such as 100% whole wheat, rye, pumpernickel, oatmeal bread, cornbread (made from whole, ground cornmeal) and bran muffins.

3. Choose whole fresh fruits and vegetables (with the skin) more often than juices.

4. Add baked beans, dried beans and peas to the menu 2-3 times per week; try adding bean soup, bean salads and hummus to the menu.

5. Choose high fiber snacks such as fresh fruit, raw vegetables, and nuts, or sprinkle unprocessed bran on yogurt for residents on mechanically altered diets. Offer stewed, dried fruits, date or fig spread on whole wheat bread or crackers, or any of the fiber-supplemented cookies or bars. Refer to the appendix for Fiber Content of Common Foods.

The National Cancer Institute and the Academy of Nutrition and Dietetics recommend a daily fiber intake of 20-35 grams of fiber per day. A wide variety of foods should be used to increase fiber intake. Encourage fluid intake of eight cups per day. Gradually increasing fiber intake is recommended to prevent cramping, abdominal distention and flatulence.

II. **Approximate Composition**
III. Calories   1600-2000
    Protein   60-75 grams
    Fiber   20-35 grams

Adequacy
This diet contains all nutrients necessary to provide and maintain adequate nutrition based on the Dietary Guidelines for Americans 2010.

*The avoidance of foods with nuts, seeds and a high content of cellulose and lignin (e.g. corn, popcorn) is recommended for diverticulitis.

Sample Menu Plan
Breakfast

Juice	Orange juice	4 ounces
Fruit	Prunes	3
Cereal	Oatmeal with bran	½ cup
Meat or equivalent	Egg, scrambled	1
Bread	Toast, whole wheat	1 slice
Fat	Soft margarine	1 packet
Milk	Milk, 2%	8 ounces
Beverage	of choice	6-8 ounces
Miscellaneous	Jelly	1 packet
	Sugar	2 packets
	Creamer	as desired
	Salt, Pepper	1 packet each

Lunch or Supper

Soup	Vegetable soup	6 ounces
Meat or equivalent	Tuna salad	½ cup
Salad	Tossed salad	1 cup
Fat	Italian dressing	1 ounce
Bread	Bread, whole wheat	2 slices
Dessert	Chilled peaches	½ cup
Milk	Milk, 2%	8 ounces
Beverage	of choice	6-8 ounces
Miscellaneous	Sugar	1 packet
	Creamer	as desired
	Salt, Pepper	1 packet each

Dinner

Meat or equivalent	Baked chicken breast	3 ounces
Vegetable	Carrots, cooked	½ cup
Salad	Mixed fruit salad	½ cup
Potato or equivalent	Red skinned potatoes	½ cup
Bread	Dinner roll/ whole wheat	1
Fat	Soft margarine	1 packet
Milk	Milk, 2%	1 cup
Dessert	Ice cream/oatmeal raisin cookie	½ cup/1
Beverage	of choice	6-8 ounces
Miscellaneous	Sugar	1 packet
	Salt, Pepper	1 packet each

Evening Nourishment

	Juice	4 ounces
	Graham Crackers	3 squares
	Fresh apple	1

*The avoidance of foods with nuts, seeds and a high content of cellulose and lignin (e.g. corn, popcorn) is recommended

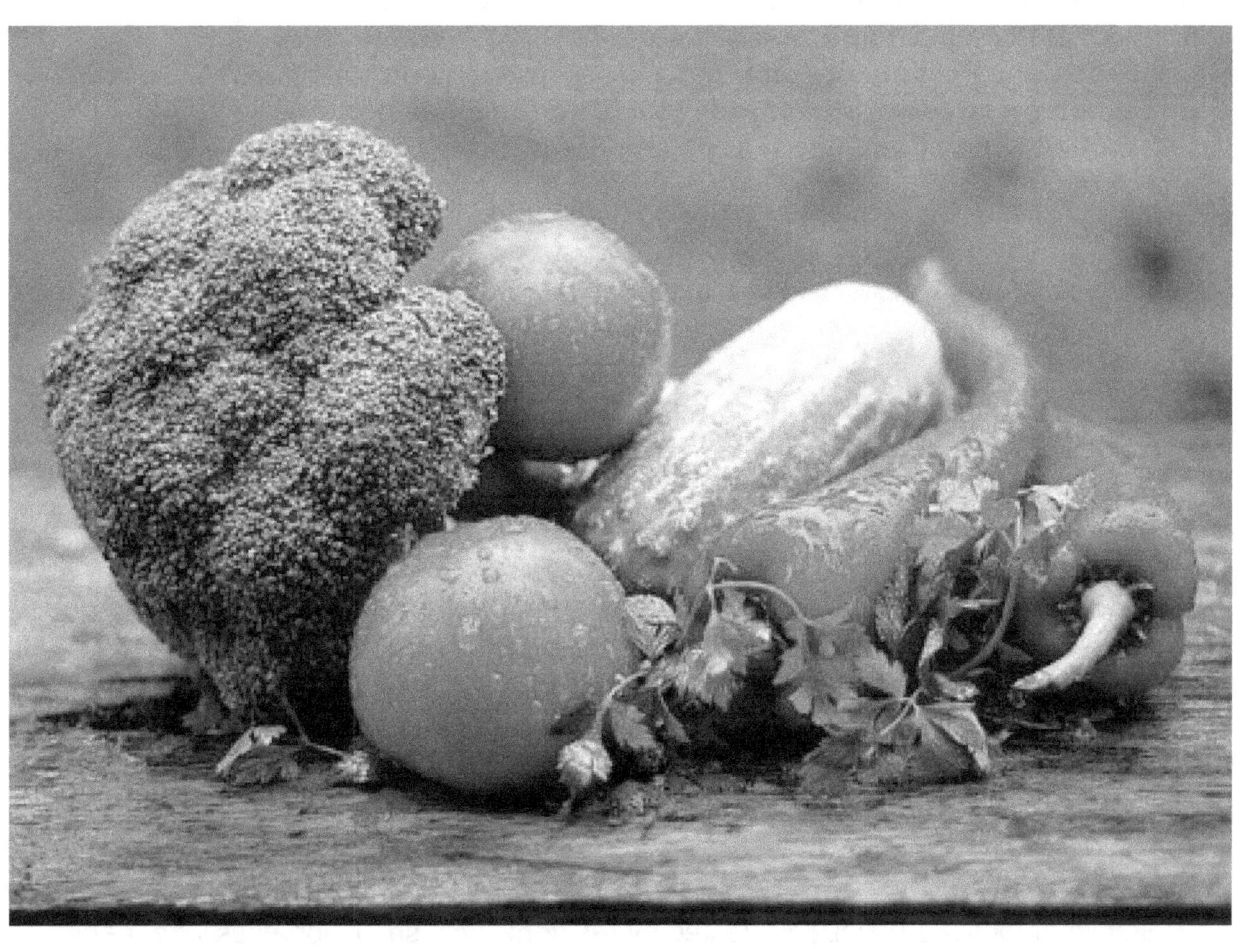

Small, Regular and Large Portion Sizes

Portion sizes may be adjusted to meet the nutritional needs and personal preferences of an individual resident. Before any adjustment is done, the dietitian should review the individual resident's nutritional needs and ascertain if the increase or decrease in portion sizes will be advantageous to the resident. Portion size changes may be warranted due to resident preferences and/or individuals on the small portion diet, multivitamin or additional supplementation may be necessary.

Food Item	Regular	Small	Large
Meats (breakfast)	1 oz.	1 oz.	2 oz.
(lunch)	3 oz.	2 oz.	4 oz.
(dinner)	3 oz.	2 oz.	4 oz.
Starches	1/2 c.	3 ¼ oz (#10)	6 oz.
Cereals -hot	1/2 c.	3 ¼ oz. (#10)	1 cup
-cold	¾ c.	¾ c.	1 1/2 c.
Vegetables	1/2 c.	3 ¼ oz. (#10)	6 oz.
Bread	1 Slice	1 Slice	1 Slice
Juice	4 oz.	4 oz.	4 oz.
Milk	8 oz.	8 oz.	8 oz.
* Fruit	½ c.	½ c.	¾ c.
* Dessert	1 svg.	1 svg.	1 svg.

Small portions are usually requested by residents with small appetites who feel overwhelmed by regular size portions or for weight control or weight reducing diet. Snacks may be needed to make up for decreased nutrient density with this diet.

* Most residents do not request small portions of these items

I. **Description**
Portion sizes may be adjusted to meet the nutritional needs and personal preferences of an individual resident. Before any adjustment is done, the dietitian will review the individual resident's nutritional needs and ascertain if the decrease in portion sizes will be advantageous to the resident. Small portions may be warranted due to resident's request and/or calorie and protein needs that are less than what the regular diet provides.

II. **Approximate Composition**
Calories   1350-1750
Protein   55-60 grams

III. **Adequacy**
This diet may be nutritionally inadequate based on the Dietary Guidelines for Americans 2010. A multivitamin or additional supplementation may be necessary.

Small Portions Diet

Sample Menu Plan
Breakfast

Fruit or juice	Orange juice	4 ounces
Cereal	Oatmeal	#10 scoop
Meat or equivalent	Scrambled egg	1 serving
Bread	Toast, whole wheat	1 slice
Fat	Soft margarine	1 packet
Milk	Milk, 2%	8 ounces
Beverage	of choice	6-8 ounces
Miscellaneous	Jelly	1 tablespoon
	Sugar	1-2 packets
	Creamer	as desired
	Salt, Pepper	1 packet each

Lunch and Supper

Meat or equivalent	Tuna salad	#10 scoop
Vegetable	Vegetable soup	6 ounces
Salad	Tossed salad	#10 scoop
Fat	Italian dressing	1 ounce
Bread	Bread, whole wheat	1 slice
Dessert	Chilled peaches	½ cup
Milk	Milk, 2%	8 ounces
Beverage	of choice	6 ounces
Miscellaneous	Sugar	1 packet
	Creamer	as desired
	Salt, Pepper	1 packet each

Meat or equivalent	Baked chicken breast	2 ounces
Starch	Mashed potatoes, gravy	#10 scoop
Fat	Soft margarine	1 packet
Vegetable	Seasoned carrots	#10 scoop
Salad	Mixed fruit	#10 scoop
Bread	Dinner roll, whole wheat	1
Milk	Milk, 2%	8 ounces
Dessert	Vanilla ice cream	½ cup
Beverage	of choice	6-8 ounces
Miscellaneous	Sugar	1 packet
	Salt, Pepper	1 packet each

Evening Nourishment

	Juice	4 ounces
	Graham crackers	3 squares

Small Portion Diet

Dinner

Sample Menu Plan

Breakfast

Fruit or juice	Orange juice	4 ounces
Cereal	Oatmeal	1 cup
Meat or equivalent	Scrambled egg	2 servings
Bread	Toast, whole wheat	1 slice
Fat	Soft margarine	1 packet
Milk	Milk, 2%	8 ounces
Beverage	of choice	6-8 ounces
Miscellaneous	Jelly	1 tablespoon
	Sugar	1-2 packets
	Creamer	as desired
	Salt, Pepper	1 packet each

Lunch/Supper

Meat or equivalent	Tuna salad	# 6 scoop
Vegetable	Vegetable soup	6 ounces
Salad	Tossed salad	1 cup
Fat	Italian dressing	2 ounces
Bread	Bread, whole wheat	1 slice
Dessert	Chilled peaches	¾ cup
Milk	Milk, 2%	8 ounces
Beverage	of choice	6 ounces
Miscellaneous	Sugar/salt/pepper	1 packet each
	Creamer	as desired

Dinner

Meat or equivalent	Baked chicken breast	4 ounces
Starch	Mashed potatoes, gravy	6 oz.
Fat	Soft Margarine	1 packet
Vegetable	Seasoned carrots	6 oz.
Fruit	Fruit Cocktail	¾ cup
Bread	Dinner roll, whole wheat	1
Milk	Milk, 2%	8 ounces
Dessert	Vanilla ice cream	½ cup
Beverage	Sugar	1 packet
Miscellaneous	Salt, Pepper	1 packet

Evening Nourishment

	Juice	4 ounces
	Graham crackers	3 squares

I. **Description**
The vegetarian diet is a modification of the regular diet. The diet is predominately composed of plant foods and may or may not include eggs and dairy. Traditionally, vegetarian diets have been classified by the type of animal products that have been excluded. These classifications include:

Lacto-ovovegetarian	Meat, poultry and fish are excluded
Lacto-vegetarian	Meat, poultry, fish and eggs are excluded
Ovovegetarian	Meat, poultry, fish, milk and milk products are excluded
Vegan	Meat, poultry, fish, eggs, milk and milk products are excluded

No matter which classification is practiced, the vegetarian diet should provide a variety of foods that ensure adequate amounts of all nutrients required for tissue repair, growth and maintenance. Careful evaluation of the resident's diet history is therefore imperative to identify the specific food practices of individual vegetarians. A variety of protein-containing foods should be planned over the course of the day to supply the amino acids needed.

The lacto-ovovegetarian diet and the vegan diet are illustrated to provide a guide to ensure nutritional adequacy.

II. **Approximate Composition**
Calories   1600 – 2000
Protein   60 – 75 grams

III. **Adequacy**
The lacto-ovovegetarian diet contains all nutrients necessary to provide and maintain adequate nutrition based on the Dietary Guidelines for Americans 2010.

The vegan diet requires special attention to ensure that all nutrients are provided. Vitamin D and Vitamin B12 may be deficient in the vegan diet. Fortified soy milk, fortified cereals and multi-vitamins with mineral supplements may be served daily to meet nutrient requirements.

Vegetarian Diet

FOOD GROUPS	FOODS INCLUDED	DAILY AMOUNT
Dairy products and (optional) dairy alternatives	All types; yogurt; soy milk fortified with calcium and Vitamin D	Up to 3 servings 1 serving equals 1 cup
Meat equivalents and (eggs, cheese optional) alternatives	Cheese: dried beans, peas, and lentils; peanut butter, nuts; tofu; soy milk; cottage cheese or ricotta; whole egg (limit egg yolks to 4 per week); egg whites and yolk free products are unlimited	At least 5 meat equivalents with 1 equivalent equaling; 1 ounce cheese or ¼ cup ricotta and cottage cheese; or 1 egg or 2 egg whites or 2 tablespoons nut butter; ¼ cup nuts; ½ cup cooked dried beans, peas and lentils; or 2 tablespoons nut butter; 4 ounces tofu; or tempeh, 1 cup soy milk
	Nuts (check nutritional analysis of individual items for amounts needed)	2 tablespoons
Fruits	All types; citrus or a high vitamin C fruit daily	3 or more servings 1 medium apple, pear, orange, banana; or ½ cup chopped, canned, cooked or frozen fruit; or ¾ cup fruit juice
Vegetables	All types, including potatoes; corn, lima beans, peas; dark green leafy or deep yellow vegetables 3-4 times a week	3 or more servings, 1 serving equals; 1 cup raw or ½ cup cooked or chopped raw; or ¾ cup juice

Vegetarian Diet

FOOD GROUPS	FOODS INCLUDED	DAILY AMOUNT
Soups	All types made with vegetable stock	As desired 1 serving equals; 6 ounces or ¾ cup
Breads, Grains & Cereals	All types, especially whole grains	6 or more servings 1 serving equals; 1 slice of bread; or ¾ - 1 ounce ready to eat cereal; or ½ cup cooked cereal; ½ cup cooked pasta or rice
Fats	All types as desired	As needed for adequate caloric intake
Desserts	All types as desired	As needed for adequate caloric intake
Beverages	All types, including at least 6 to 8 cups of water and other fluids per day	As needed to meet fluid requirements
Miscellaneous	Sugar, condiments, jelly preserves, syrup, sweets, herbs, spices, salt, and flavorings	As desired for adequate caloric intake, flavor, and palatability

Sample Menu Plan
Breakfast

Fruit or juice	Orange juice	¾ cup
Cereal	Oatmeal	1 cup
Meat equivalent	Scrambled egg	1
Bread	Whole wheat toast	1 slice
Fat	Soft Margarine	1 teaspoon
Beverage	of choice	6-8 ounces
Milk	Milk, 2%	8 ounces
Miscellaneous	Sugar	3 packets
	Creamer, non-dairy	as desired
	Salt, pepper	1 packet each

Lunch

Soup	Vegetable Soup	1 cup
Bread	Whole wheat bread	2 slices
Meat equivalent	American cheese	2 ounces
	Mayonnaise	1 tablespoon
Salad	Tossed salad	1 cup
Fat	Italian Dressing	1 ounce
Dessert	Chilled peaches	½ cup
Beverage	of choice	6-8 ounces
Milk	Milk, 2%	8 ounces
Miscellaneous	Sugar	1-3 packets
	Creamer, non dairy	as desired
	Salt, pepper	1 packet each

Evening Nourishment

	Graham cracker	3 squares
	Fruit juice	4 ounces

Dinner

Meat equivalent	Black beans	1 cup
Potato or equivalent	Brown rice	½ cup
Vegetable	Sliced carrots	½ cup
Salad	Mixed fruit salad	1 cup
Bread	Roll, whole wheat	1 l
Fat	Soft margarine	1 teaspoon
Dessert	Vanilla ice cream	½ cup
Beverage	of choice	6-8 ounces
Milk	Milk, 2%	1 cup
Miscellaneous	Sugar	1-2 packets
	Creamer, non-dairy	as desired
	Salt, pepper	1 packet each

Vegan Meal Plan

Sample Menu Plan

Breakfast

Fruit or juice	Orange juice	¾ cup
Cereal	Oatmeal – prepared with soy milk	1 cup
Meat equivalent	Peanut butter	2 tablespoons
Bread	Whole wheat toast	1 slice
Fat	Soft margarine	1 teaspoon
Beverage	Coffee	6 ounces
	Ice water	8 ounces
Milk Equivalent	Soy milk	1 cup
Miscellaneous	Sugar	3 packets
	Creamer, non-dairy	2 packets
	Salt, pepper	1 packet each

Lunch

Meat equivalent	Black beans	1 cup
Potato or equivalent	Brown rice	½ cup
Salad	Vegetable soup	1 cup
	Tossed salad	1 cup
	Italian Dressing	1 ounce
Bread	Bread, whole wheat	1 slice
Fat	Soft margarine	1 packet
Dessert	Chilled peaches	½ cup
Beverage	of choice	6-8 ounces
Miscellaneous	Sugar	1-3 packets
	Salt, pepper	1 packet each
Evening Nourishment	Graham crackers	3 squares
	Fruit juice	4 ounces

Dinner

Meat equivalent	Tofu	1 cup
Vegetable	Sliced carrots	½ cup
Salad	Citrus section salad	½ cup
Bread	Dinner roll, whole wheat	1 slice
Fat	Soft margarine	1 packet
Dessert	Cherry gelatin	1 cup
Beverage	of choice	6-8 ounces
	Soy milk	1 cup
Miscellaneous	Sugar	1-2 packets
	Creamer, non-dairy	2 packets
Salt, pepper	1 packet each	

No Added Salt (NAS) Diet

This diet is a regular diet with the exception that no salt may be added to food after preparation. No salt is allowed with the resident's meals. Salt substitute should be used only with a physician's order.

Low Sodium Diet (2-4 grams)

I. **Description**

This diet may be used to help control mild hypertension or edema. It may be effective when used in conjunction with drug therapy when either condition is more severe but a stricter diet regime is not feasible. The FOODS INCLUDED on this diet are similar to that of a regular diet, with the omission of highly salted foods and table salt.

The following guidelines are used for planning and preparation of the diet.

1. Use a moderate* amount of salt in cooking but serve no salt on the tray.
2. Avoid highly salted foods such as bouillon, soup and gravy bases, canned soups and stews; bread and rolls with salted toppings, salted crackers; salted nuts, popcorn, potato chips, pretzels, and other salted snacks. (Reduced sodium products may be used, check label).
3. Avoid all salt cured, smoked and processed smoked meats, such as ham, bacon, cold cuts, chipped and corned beef, frankfurters, Koshered or Kosher style meats; canned meat and poultry. (Reduced sodium products may be used; check label.)
4. Avoid salted and smoked fish, such as cod, herring, sardines; canned salted salmon and tuna.
5. Avoid sauerkraut, olives, pickles, relishes, and other vegetables prepared in brine; tomato and vegetable cocktail juices canned with salt.
6. Avoid seasonings such as celery salt, garlic salt, Worcestershire sauce, soy sauce, and others containing salt; no salt substitutes unless ordered by the physician.
7. Serve cheeses, e.g., cheddar, mozzarella, provolone, and processed cheeses such as American, in limited amounts (approximately two times a week) unless low sodium (read labels).

II. **Approximate Composition**
   Calories   1600-2000
   Protein   60-75 grams
   Sodium   2-4 grams

III. **Adequacy**

This diet contains all nutrients necessary to provide and maintain adequate nutrition based on the Dietary Reference Intakes-2005 Revision.

*A moderate amount of salt is the amount usually called for in a standardized recipe. If no salt is used in the cooking, the sodium content of the diet may be below 2 grams.

Cholesterol Restricted and Fat Controlled Diet

I. Description

This diet is designed to limit total fat, saturated fat, and cholesterol intake. The intent is to reduce and maintain an acceptable blood cholesterol level for the resident. This diet may also be used for disorders of the gall bladder, pancreas, and liver. The American Heart Association recommends total fat be no more than 20-25 percent of the total daily calories, with saturated fat limited to approximately 10 percent of total fat. The American Heart Association recommends limiting the amount of trans fats you eat to less than one percent of your total daily calories. That means if you need 2000 calories a day, no more than 20 of those calories should come from trans fats. That is less than 2 grams of trans fat a day.

There are "low fat" and "fat free" products currently available which are suitable for use on this diet and which may not be identified here. Read labels carefully to verify the appropriateness of the product(s) for use.

Fat Free – no more than 0.5 grams of fat per standardized serving
Low fat – no more than 3 grams of fat per standardized serving
Low saturated fat – no more than 1 gram of saturated fat per standardized serving
Low cholesterol – no more than 20 milligrams of cholesterol per standardized serving

II. Approximate Composition

Calories   1600-2000
Protein   60-75 grams
Cholesterol   300 milligrams

III. Adequacy

This diet provides all nutrients necessary to provide and maintain adequate nutrition based on the Dietary Guidelines for Americans 2010.

Cholesterol Restricted and Fat Controlled Diet

FOOD GROUPS	FOODS INCLUDED	FOODS EXCLUDED
Milk	1% Skim, buttermilk and lowfat yogurt and milk	All others including whole milk, 2% Milk products
Meat and equivalents	Limit to 6 ounces per day: lean beef, veal, lamb and pork, crab, shrimp, lobster and oysters. Select from the following for other meats: chicken and turkey without skin; fish, including canned water packed salmon and tuna; peanut butter in limited amounts, lowfat cold cuts; meats, poultry and fish should be baked, broiled, roasted, simmered, or steamed and all visible fat removed	Marbled or fatty meats; fried or sautéed; Skin of chicken and turkey; duck; goose; fish canned in oil; regular luncheon meats; canned meats; salt pork, frankfurters and hot dogs; bacon;
	Low fat cheeses; ricotta and cottage cheese;	Other cheeses, dips, and spreads
	Eggs, cooked, without additional fat (limit egg yolks to 3 per week); without additional fat and in cooking. Unlimited cholesterol free egg products; dried beans, peas, and lentils.	Eggs, prepared with additional fat

Seasoned with any food not allowed |

Cholesterol Restricted and Fat Controlled Diet

FOOD GROUPS	FOODS INCLUDED	FOODS EXCLUDED
Fruits	All types	None
Vegetables	All types	Any prepared with bacon, meat drippings, butter, cream, whole or 2% milk
Soup	Bouillon, consommé, clear broth; soups made with fat free broth or skim milk	All others
Breads, Cereals & Grains	All types including noodles, pasta and rice; waffles and pancakes;	Sweet rolls, quick breads; (muffins, biscuits, cornbread), doughnuts
Fats	Use sparingly	Saturated fats such as butter, cream, bacon, shortening; oils; high fat salad dressing.
Desserts	Lowfat cake, pudding, fruit and cream pie and ice cream; cookies gelatin; sherbet; fruit whips; water ice;	High fat desserts
Beverages	Carbonated beverages, coffee, tea, fruit drinks	All others
Miscellaneous	Sugar, condiments, jam, jelly, preserves, syrup, honey, hard candy, gum drops, jelly beans, marshmallows	Chocolate candy; baking chocolate

Cholesterol Restricted and Fat Controlled Diet

Sample Menu Plan

Breakfast

Fruit or juice	Orange juice	4 ounces
Cereal	Oatmeal	½ cup
Meat equivalent	Cholesterol free egg	1
Bread	Toast whole wheat	1 slice
Fat	Soft margarine	1 teaspoon
Beverage	of choice	6-8 ounces
Milk	Skim milk	8 ounces
Miscellaneous	Jelly	1 packet
	Sugar	2 packets
	Creamer	as desired
	Salt, pepper	1 packet each

Lunch or Supper

Meat equivalent	Tuna salad	½ cup
Vegetable	Vegetable soup	6 ounces
Salad	Tossed salad	1 cup
Fat	Lowfat Italian dressing	1 ounce
Bread	Whole wheat bread	2 slices
Dessert	Chilled peaches	½ cup
Milk	Skim milk	8 ounces
Beverage	of choice	6-8 ounces
Miscellaneous	Sugar	1-2 packets
	Creamer	as desired
	Salt, pepper	1 packet each

Dinner

Meat equivalent	Baked chicken breast	½ (3 ounces EP) (without skin)
Potato	Mashed potatoes	½ cup
	low fat gravy	1 ounce
Vegetable	Seasoned carrots	½ cup
Salad	Mixed fruit salad	½ cup
Bread	Dinner roll, whole wheat	1
Fat	Soft margarine	1 teaspoons
Milk	Skim milk	8 ounces
Dessert	Rainbow sherbet	½ cup
Beverage	of choice	6-8 ounces
Miscellaneous	Sugar	1-2 packets
	Creamer	as desired
	Salt, Pepper	1 packet each

Evening Nourishment

	Juice	8 ounces
	Graham crackers	3 squares

Limited K+ Diet

Avoid the following foods and beverages;

- Bananas
- Prunes and prune juice
- Orange Juice
- Baked potatoes and sweet potatoes
- Tomatoes, tomato juice, V-8 juice

Encourage the following lower k+ beverage choices in addition to water:

- Cranberry juice
- Lemonade
- Apple juice
- Grape juice
- Fruit punch
- Clear soda

Liberalized Renal Diet

Follow K+ guidelines above

Limit obviously salted foods

- Meats: sausage, bacon, scrapple, ham, chipped beef, corned beef, hot dogs, Canned meats
- Potato chips, salty snack foods
- Pickles, olives, sauerkraut

Renal Diet

I. **Description**

This diet is designed for residents with acute or chronic renal failure.

There are two categories of the Renal Diet including:

1. A predialysis diet in which the purpose is to restrict the intake of protein and phosphorus, potassium, sodium and fluid as medically indicated.
2. A dialysis diet is a liberalized and less restrictive diet. This diet is used to encourage the resident to improve their oral intake and help prevent malnutrition.

The renal diet order for potassium and sodium is usually written in milliEquivalents (mEq) but the food content of these minerals is generally given in milligrams (mg). To convert one measure to the other, see the appendix (page 122).

When planning a renal diet, the Carbohydrate Control Exchange Lists should be used. The pattern for each resident should be planned according to individual needs including labs, weights and preferences. Four commonly ordered renal diets are included that can be used as guides in planning menus.

II. **Approximate Composition**

	Predialysis	**Dialysis**
Calories	2000	2000
Protein	45 gram (gm)	75 gm
Potassium (K)	As medically indicated	As medically indicated
Sodium (Na)	2-4 gm Na	2-4 gm Na
Phosphorus (PO4)	850 mg 1000 mg	less than 1700 mg
Fluid (ml/d)	As medically indicated	As medically indicated

III. **Adequacy**

The 45 gm protein diet is deficient in thiamine, riboflavin, niacin, calcium, vitamin C, vitamin D, vitamin A, copper, magnesium, zinc and iron based on the Dietary Guidelines for Americans 2010.

The 60 gram protein diet is inadequate in calcium, pantothenic acid, copper, vitamin A, vitamin B6, magnesium and zinc based on the Dietary Guidelines for Americans 2010.

In addition, the patient who is receiving hemodialysis treatment will lose water soluble vitamins during dialysis.

Renal Diet
Protein Levels*

	45 grams	60 grams	75 grams	90 grams
Breakfast				
Whole Milk	½ cup	1 cup	1 cup	1 cup
Egg	1	1	1	1
Starch	2	2	2	3
Fruit	1	1	1	1
Fat	2	2	3	3
Lunch				
Meat	1	2	3	3
Starch	2	2	2	2
Vegetable	1	1	1	1
Fruit	1	1	1	1
Fat	3	3	3	3
Dinner				
Meat	1	1	2	3
Starch	2	2	2	2
Vegetable	1	1	1	1
Fruit	1	1	1	1
Fat	3	3	3	3
Evening Snack				
Fruit	1	1	1	1
Starch	1	1	1	1
Meat	0	0	0	1
Fat	0	0	0	1

*follows carbohydrate control exchange list
**protein needs are increased for the resident undergoing dialysis

Renal Diet
Fluid Restriction Distribution Guide

This guide is to be followed until an individualized plan is developed by the dietitian and/or nursing service along with the resident's input. It is suggested to use applesauce for the administration of medications.

Anything liquid at room temperature should be considered a liquid, eg: ice cream, gelatin, sherbet, popsicle, syrup, gravy, juice in canned fruits.
KEEP NO WATER CUP AT THE BEDSIDE (unless ordered by physician).

120 ml = 1/2 cup   240 ml = 1 cup

TYPE	AMOUNT OF FLUID IN ml				
BREAKFAST					
Juice	120	120	120	240	240
Beverage	120	240	240	240	240
NOON MEAL					
Beverage	120	240	240	240	240
EVENING MEAL					
Milk	120	120	120	240	240
Beverage	120	120	240	240	240
HS SNACK					
Milk	120	120			
Juice			120	120	240
FROM NURSING	280	240	420	480	560
TOTAL FLUIDS IN 24 HOURS	1000	1200	1500	1800	2000

Potassium (K) mg

Items	Serving	Mg K+
FRUITS & JUICES		
Apricots, fresh	3 medium	313
Apricots dried halves	10 each	482
Avocado-California	1 med	1097
Florida	1 med	1484
Banana	1 med	451
Blackberry juice	1 cup	425
Cantaloupe, cubes	1 cup	494
Cherries, sweet, fresh, pitted	1 cup	325
Dates, whole, pitted	10 ea	541
Grape Juice, canned/bottled	1 cup	334
Grapefruit, half, canned sections	1 cup	328
Grapefruit juice, fresh	1 cup	400
Prepared from frozen	1 cup	337
Canned unsweetened	1 cup	378
Canned sweetened	1 cup	405
Honeydew Melon, cubes	1 cup	461
Lemon Juice: Fresh	1 cup	303
Melon Casaba Cubes	1 cup	357
Orange Juices		
Chilled, fresh	1 cup	473
Prep. From frozen	1 cup	474
Canned, unsweetened	1 cup	436
Orange Grapefruit juice	1 cup	390
Papaya	1 each	780
Passion fruit juice		
Purple	1 cup	343
Yellow	1 cup	687
Plantains, cooked	1 cup	716
Pineapple Juice	1 cup	338
Pomegranate	1 ea	399
Prunes, dried	10 ea	626
Prune juice	1 cup	707
Raisins	1 cup	1089
Rhubarb, fresh	1 cup	351
VEGETABLES		
Artichoke, hearts marinated	6 oz	438
Asparagus, frozen	1 cup	392
Bamboo shoots, cooked fresh	1 cup	640
Baked beans, dry white w/sauce	1 cup	907

Black Beans	1 cup	611
Black eyed peas, cooked from froz	1 cup	860
Cooked from fresh	1 cup	690
Canned	1 cup	413
Cooked from dry	1 cup	476
Bok choy, fresh cooked	1 cup	630
Broad bean, canned	1 cup	620
Broccoli		
Fresh chopped, cooked	1 cup	456
Frozen, cooked	1 cup	331
Brussel sprouts		
frozen cooked	1 cup	504
Fresh cooked	1 cup	491
Cabbage cooked	1 cup	308
Carrot juice	½ cup	358
Celery, cooked, fresh	1 cup	426
Chard, Swiss fresh -cooked	1 cup	961
Collards, cooked from frozen	1 cup	307
Eggplant, fresh cooked	1 cup	397
Garbanzo beans, dry cooked	1 cup	477
Great Northern beans, dry cooked	1 cup	692
Green (snap) beans, cooked fresh	1 cup	373
Green peas, cooked fresh	1 cup	383
Hyacinth Beans, cooked, dry	1 cup	653
Kale, cooked from frozen	1 cup	417
Kidney beans, canned	1 cup	658
Cooked from dry	1 cup	713
Kohlrabi fresh	1 cup	490
Cooked	1 cup	561
Lentils, Cooked from dry	1 cup	731
Lotus root, cooked fresh	10 each	323
Parsnips, cooked from fresh	1 cup	573
POTATOES: (unless leached)		
Chips	14 chips = 1 oz	369
Baked, Flesh & skin	1 each	844
Flesh only	1 each	610
Potato Skin	1 each	332
Boiled w/skin, flesh only	1 each	515
French Fries, fried in oil	10 each	366
Hash browns, Frozen	1 cup	680
Mashed, w/milk/marg	1 cup	607
Prepared w/milk	1 cup	628
From instant	1 cup	428
Pumpkin, mashed, fresh	1 cup	564

Rutabaga, fresh cubed	1 cup	471
Sauerkraut, canned	1 cup	401
Soybeans, dry cooked	1 cup	886
Spinach, frozen cooked	1 cup	566
Fresh cooked	1 cup	838
Fresh	1 cup	312
Canned, drained	1 cup	740
Squash, Summer, sliced		
Crookneck, fresh cooked	1 cup	346
Zucchini, cooked fresh	1 cup	455
Winter Squash		
Acorn (Danish), baked	1 cup	1071
Butternut, baked	1 cup	697
Hubbard, baked	1 cup	859
Succotash, cooked from fresh	1 cup	757
Frozen cooked	1 cup	451
Sweet potatoes, baked	1 cup	397
Taro, fresh	1 cup	615
TOMOTOES:		
Fresh chopped	1 cup	400
Cooked from fresh	1 cup	670
Juice	1 cup	537
Paste	1 cup	2442
Sauce	1 cup	908
Puree	1 cup	1051
Mixed Vegetables (corn, peas, Limas, green beans, carrots) frozen, cooked	1 cup	308
Canned, drained	1 cup	474
MILK & DAIRY		
CHEESE:		
Ricotta, part skim	1 cup	307
CREAM, Sweet fluid,		
Half & Half	1 cup	314
CREAM, sour		
Cultured dairy	1 cup	331
Imitation non-dairy	1 cup	369
CREAM SUBSTITUTES, non dairy		
Coffee whitener (powder)	1 cup	763
MILK		
Skim	1 cup	406
Lowfat 1 %	1 cup	381
Lowfat 2 %	1 cup	377
Whole (3.3% fat)	1 cup	370
Buttermilk (<1% fat)	1 cup	371
Canned, skim evap	1 cup	845
Canned, whole	1 cup	764
Dry, instant nonfat, envelope	1 each	1552

	Dried, buttermilk	1 cup	1910
Milk (other):			
	Goat	1 cup	499
	Soy Milk	1 cup	338
Chocolate			
	Low fat 1%	1 cup	425
	Low fat 1 %	1 cup	422
	Whole (3.3 % fat)	1 cup	417
Egg Nog, commercial		1 cup	420
Malted Milk, w/whole milk			
	Chocolate flavor	1 cup	499
	Natural Flavor	1 cup	529
Milkshakes 10 Fl Oz, 1.25 c			
	Chocolate	1.25 cup	567
	Strawberry	1.25 cup	516
	Vanilla	1.25 cup	492
MILK DESSERTS:			
	Custard Baked	1 cup	387
	Soft Served ice cream, vanilla	1 cup	338
	Ice milk soft serve 3 %fat	1 cup	412
Chocolate Pudding		1 cup	366
YOGURT			
	Lowfat plain	1 cup	531
	Lowfat w/fruit	1 cup	442
	Lowfat, coffee/vanilla	1 cup	497
	Nonfat	1 cup	579
	Whole	1 cup	352
	Yogurt, cheese	1 cup	666
MEAT, FISH & POULTRY			
BEEF			
	Rib, lean only, roasted	3 ounces	320
	Round Steak, lean only broiled	3 ounces	352
	Round Steak, lean & fat broiled	3 ounces	311
	Round tip lean only, roasted	3 ounces	328
	Sirloin Steak, lean only, broiled	3 ounces	336
	T-Bone Steak, lean only broiled	3 ounces	346
	Beef fried liver	3 ounces	309

PORK		
Center loin chop broiled lean, & fat, (cut 3 per lb = 4.4 oz-raw w/o bone, 5.3 oz-raw w/bone)		
Broiled, lean & fat	1 each	312
Broiled, lean only	1 each	302
Pan fried, lean & fat, center	1 each	323
Pan fried, lean only	1 each	305
Center rib chop: (cut 3 per lb, 5.3 oz raw w/bone 3.9 oz w/o bone)		
Pan Fried, lean & fat	1 each	309
Pork roast, leg, lean only	3 ounces	317
Pork roast, average loin & rib, lean only	3 ounces	333
Spare ribs, cooked 1 lb raw	6.25 oz	566
Veal (calf) liver, pan fried	3 ounces	372
POULTRY:		
CHICKEN: 3 lb = 1.45 lb raw, =1.1 lb cooked		
Fried	1 cup	360
Roasted	1 cup	340
Goose, domestic Roasted Meat only	3 oz	330
TURKEY:		
Roasted all types	1 cup	418
Sausages and Lunchmeats		
Ham Salad Spread	1 cup	359
Grains & Grain Products:		
Amaranth grain	1 cup	714
Buckwheat Flour, dark	1 cup	490
Buckwheat Flour, light	1 cup	314
Corn Flour	1 cup	369
Masa Harina, enriched	1 cup	340

Cornmeal, dry:		
Nearly whole broiled	1 cup	303
FLOUR:		
Macaroni, cooked:		
Vegetable enriched	1 cup	413
NOODLES:		
Oat bran (1 T = 6g)	1 cup	532
PASTA:		
Quinoa grain, dry	1 cup	1258
RICE, cooked:		
Rice bran	1 cup	1233
Rye Flour, Dark	1 cup	934
Soy Flour, stirred:		
Low fat flour	½ cup	1131
Defatted	½ cup	1192
Full fat, raw	½ cup	1069
WHEAT:		
Wheat bran	½ cup	355
FLOURS, unbleached		
Semolina	1 cup	311
Whole Wheat	1 cup	486
Wheat Germ		
Raw	1 cup	892
Toasted	1 cup	1070
Wheat, rolled, dry	1 cup	323
MIXED DISHES & FAST FOODS		
Beef & Vegetable stew		
Recipe	1 cup	613
Canned	1 cup	417
Beef, macaroni, tomato Sauce,		
Recipe	1 cup	562
Beef Pot Pie, homemade	1 piece	334
BURRITO		
Bean Burrito	1 each	427
Beef Burrito	1 each	363
Beef & Bean Burrito	1 each	388
Deluxe Combination	1 each	433
Chicken a la king, recipe	1 cup	404
Chicken Chow Mein		
Homemade	1 cup	473
Canned	1 cup	418
Chicken curry, homemade	1.5 cup	410
Chicken pot pie, recipe, 1/3	1 piece	343
Chili w/beans, canned	1 cup	932
Chop suey, beef/pork	1 cup	425
Corn pudding	1 cup	402

Corned beef hash, canned	1 cup	440
LASAGNA, recipe		
with meat	1 piece	507
without meat	1 piece	424
Manicotti, frozen entree	1 each	347
Moussaka (lamb & eggplant)	1 cup	695
PIZZA, cheese		
Regular crust, 1/8 of 15"	1 piece	474
Thick crust, ½ of 10	1 piece	367
Potato salad w/mayo & eggs	1 cup	635
Ravioli, beef, canned = 16/cup	1 cup	553
SANDWICHES, Fast Food		
Cheeseburger, 4 oz beef	1 each	407
Fish Sandwich		
Large, w/o cheese	1 each	375
Hamburger, 4 oz beef	1 each	404
Roast beef w/bun	1 each	338
SANDWICHES, on part whole Wheat bread, unless stated as rye		
Avocado, cheese, tomato, sprouts	1 each	562
Ham & Cheese	1 each	334
Ham & Swiss on rye	1 each	342
Ham on rye	1 each	311
Patty melt, on rye	1 each	410
Reuben, grilled	1 each	313
Roast beef sandwich	1 each	314
Turkey ham & cheese on rye	1 each	319
SPAGHETTI, pasta & tomato Sauce with cheese		
Homemade	1 cup	408
Canned	1 cup	303
SPAGHETTI, pasta & tomato Sauce w/meat:		
Homemade	1 cup	665
Tostada:		
Beans & Beef	1 each	442
Beans & chicken	1 each	358
Refried Beans	1 each	422
Tuna salad	1 each	531

NUTS & SEEDS		
Almonds dried whole	1 cup	1034
Brazil nuts, dry	1 cup	840
Cashews		
Dry roasted	1 cup	774
Oil roasted	1 cup	689
Chestnuts, roasted	1 cup	846
Coconut:		
Dried, unsweetened	1 cup	423
Coconut cream, raw	1 cup	780
Coconut milk, canned	1 cup	497
Coconut water, raw	1 cup	600
Filberts (hazelnuts), whole	1 cup	601
Macadamias, oil roasted	1 cup	441
MIXED NUTS w/peanuts (almonds, brazil nuts, cashews, Filberts, peanuts & pecans)		
Dry roasted	1 cup	817
Oil roasted	1 cup	825
MIXED NUTS w/o peanuts (cashews, almonds, brazil nuts, Pecans & filberts:		
Oil roasted	1 cup	783
PEANUTS:		
Dry roasted	1 cup	960
Oil roasted	1 cup	982
Pecans, dried, chopped	1 cup	466
Pistachios, dried, shelled	1 cup	1399
Pumpkin seed		
Roasted kernels	1 cup	1830
Whole, roasted	1 cup	588
Sesame Seeds:		
Whole seed, dried	1 cup	674
Kernels, dried	1 cup	611
Soybeans, roasted	½ cup	1264
Sunflower seed kernels:		
Dried seeds	1 cup	992
Oil roasted	1 cup	652
Walnuts, chopped:		
Black	1 cup	655
English	1 cup	602

Cheese sauce: mix with milk	1 cup	552
Spaghetti sauce, plain:		
Homemade	1 cup	915
Canned	1 cup	957
Spaghetti sauce, w/meat:		
Homemade	1 cup	615
Canned	1 cup	444
White sauce		
Recipe, medium	1 cup	381
Mix with milk	1 cup	444
SOUPS: soups are prepared From canned unless Otherwise stated. RTS = Ready to serve. For Soup Prep. w/milk, assume whole Milk.		
Bean w/bacon	1 cup	403
Celery, cream of, w/milk	1 cup	309
Cheese soup w/milk	1 cup	340
Chili beef	1 cup	525
Clam chowder		
New England style	1 cup	300
Gazpacho soup, RTS	1 cup	356
Lentil & Ham RTS	1 cup	356
Minestrone soup	1 cup	312
Potato, cream of, w/milk	1 cup	323
Split pea	1 cup	399
Tomato Soup		
Prep with milk	1 cup	450
Tomato Rice Soup	1 cup	330
Turkey soup, chunky, RTS	1 cup	814
Vegetable, chunky, RTS	1 cup	396
OTHER		
Cooking ingredients, Condiments, fat, flavorings, Spices, sweets, etc		
Baking powder, low sodium	1 tsp	471
Barbecue sauce	1 cup	435
Candy and Candy bars: Chocolate coated:		
Almonds	1 cup	1011
Peanuts	1 cup	857
Raisins	1 cup	1153
Carob Flour	1 cup	852
Chili sauce:		
Tomato based	1 cup	1010
Chocolate:		

Cocoa Powder	1 cup	1000
Hummous	1 cup	427
Molasses:		
Blackstrap	2 T	1171
Natto (Soybean products)	½ cup	1276
Salt substitutes vary, check label		
Lite Salt (Morton)	1 tsp	1500
Salt Substitiute (Morton)	1 tsp	2800
Seasoned Salt Substitute (Morton)	1 tsp	2100
Sugar		
Brown	1 cup	757
SPICES		
Cream of tartar	1 T	361
Tempeh (soybean product)	1 T	609
BAKED GOODS PIE: piece is 1/16 th of 9 " pie		
Mincemeat pie	1 piece	349
Pumkin pie	1 piece	400
Banana Cream, commercial	1 piece	308
EGGS		
Egg substitutes vary by brand. Check label	1 cup	
Liquid	1 cup	828

For fresh potatoes (white or sweet) peel, slice and soak in cold water at least 4 hours (preferably overnight) drain, add fresh water and cook. Use no more than 2 times per week.

High Phosphorus Foods

These foods may need to be limited when planning a renal diet.

MILK PRODUCTS
(limit to 1 serving/day)
- 1 oz Cheese
- ½ cup Cream soup
- 1 tbsp Creamer half and half
- ½ cup Ice cream, ice milk
- ½ cup Milk
- ½ cup Milk shakes
- ½ cup Pudding
- ½ cup Yogurt

NUTS AND SEEDS
- 1 oz Almonds
- 1 oz Cashews
- 1 oz Peanuts
- 2 tbsp Peanut butter
- 1 oz Pecans
- 1 oz Pumpkin seeds
- *1 oz Sunflower seeds
- 1 oz Walnuts

GRAIN PRODUCTS
- 1 Biscuit from mix
- * ¾ cup Bran cereals
- 1 Bran muffins
- 1 Cornbread
- ½ cup Oatmeal
- 2 pancakes from mix
- 1 slice Pumpernickel bread
- 1 Waffles, except Eggo's (not banana or oats)
- 1 Whole wheat bread

MISCELLANEOUS
- Beer
- *1 cup Cocoa made with milk
- 1 oz Chocolate, semi sweet
- 12 oz Cola

LEGUMES
- ½ cup baked beans
- ½ cup Black-eyed peas
- ½ cup Chick peas (garbanzo beans)
- ½ cup Lentils
- ½ cup Lima beans
- ½ cup Navy beans
- ½ cup Red kidney beans
- *½ cup Soybean products
- *½ cup Tofu, raw, firm

PROTEIN FOODS
- *3 oz liver
- *1 oz macaroni and cheese
- *1 slice Pizza
- *3 oz Tuna
- *3 oz Salmon
- *3 oz Beef, Turkey or Ham

*These foods have greater than 200 mg of phosphorus per serving size noted. It is important to adhere to the portion sizes listed and follow the Renal Diet Pattern.

Renal Diet

I. Suggested bag lunch when sending your resident out prior to the facility lunch meal; choose a sandwich, beverage and fruit from the following list and add additional items based on need and preference.

II. Sensible Snack Suggestion

SANDWICHES

Roast beef, meat loaf, sliced chicken, sliced turkey, chicken salad, tuna, salad, seafood salad, egg salad, turkey salad, roast pork, jelly or cream cheese.

BEVERAGES

Cranberry drink, apple juice, grape juice, Hi-C, Hawaiian punch, Kool-aid, Tang, clear soda

DESSERTS

Rice crispy bar, 4 sugar cookies, 3 butter cookies, 3 vanilla cream cookies, angel food cake, pound cake, 4 shortbread cookies, fruit pie, 3 gingersnaps, or 4 vanilla wafers

FRUIT

Applesauce, apple, tangerine, grapes, blueberries, cherries, strawberries, canned pears or canned pineapple

STARCHES

Bagel with cream cheese and jelly, muffin with margarine and jelly, Danish, donut, tortilla chips, graham crackers with cream cheese, unsalted popcorn, unsalted crackers and pretzels

CANDY

Gum drops, jelly beans, hard candy, marshmallows, lollipops, candy corn or butter mints

Simplified Guideline for Standard Carbohydrate Controlled Diet

I. **Description**
Because of the importance of proper diet in the treatment and control of diabetes, whenever possible the carbohydrate controlled diet should be created by a registered or licensed dietitian/nutritionist to assure optimal variety, client satisfaction and therapeutic benefit. However, the following guideline can be used to prepare a more standard carbohydrate controlled menu. It can be used by caregivers responsible for preparing carbohydrate controlled menus in smaller assisted living programs. Once written, these menus should then be reviewed and approved by a registered/licensed dietitian/nutritionist.

II. **Approximate Composition**
The accepted calorie range for the regular diet (upon which the carbohydrate controlled diet is based) is 1700-2400 calories per day. Therefore, these simplified guidelines are designed to create a menu plan providing approximately 2000-2100 calories, 75 grams of protein, 270 grams of carbohydrate and 50 grams of fat. (Note: Calculations are based upon the use of primarily leaner meats and reduced fat (2%) milk. However, the use of whole milk is acceptable.

III. **Adequacy**
This diet contains all nutrients necessary to provide and maintain adequate nutrition based on the Recommended Daily Intakes (RDI), 2005.

IV. **Suggested Guidelines**
The diet will provide three meals and one bedtime snack daily. By using the following guidelines, the carbohydrate is distributed in equal amounts across breakfast, lunch and dinner, with a smaller amount provided at the bedtime snack.

Breakfast	Lunch	Dinner	Bedtime
3 starch servings	4 starch servings	3 starch servings	1 starch serving
1 fruit serving	1 fruit serving	1 fruit serving	1 fruit serving
	1 vegetable serving	2 vegetable serving	
1 milk serving		1 milk serving	
1 oz meat or substitute	3 oz meat or substitute	3 oz meat or substitute	1 oz meat or substitute
1 fat serving	1 fat serving	1 fat serving	1 fat serving

Simplified Guideline for Standard Carbohydrate Controlled Diet

In general, one starch serving is:
½ cup of cereal grain, pasta, or starchy vegetable, 1 ounce of a bread product, such as 1 slice of bread or crackers

In general, on fruit serving is:
1 small to medium fresh fruit
½ cup canned or fresh fruit or juice
¼ cup dried fruit

In general, one vegetable serving is:
½ cup of cooked vegetables,
1 cup vegetable juice or
1 cup raw vegetables

In general, 1 oz. meat or substitute is:
1 oz meat, poultry, fish or cheese
1 egg or ¼ cup cottage cheese
½ cup beans, peas, lentils (also count as one starch)
2 tablespoon salad dressing

See the Exchange Lists for Meal Planning at the end of this section for more detail.

Carbohydrate Controlled Diet

I. **Description**
This diet is designed for residents with diabetes mellitus. It is based upon the regular diet but, since the carbohydrate content of meals produces the largest influence on blood sugar levels, meals are planned to provide a consistent amount of carbohydrate from day to day. Concentrated sweets are not prohibited but must be planned into the total carbohydrate allowance. This diet can be used for any diabetic resident who does not require a calorie restriction.

II. **Approximate**
Calories   1700-2400
Protein   65-75 grams

III. **Adequacy**
This diet contains all nutrients necessary to provide and maintain adequate nutrition based on the Dietary Guidelines for Americans 2010.

IV. **Basis for Calculation of Carbohydrates**
The carbohydrate controlled diet is most easily planned by using the Exchange Lists for Meal Planning. There are four food exchange groups which contain carbohydrate; these are starches, fruits, milks and vegetables. In the 1994 revision to the exchange lists, another group called "other carbohydrates" was added to accommodate carbohydrate-containing foods which cannot be categorized as a starch, fruit, milk or vegetable. Examples are sweets and high fat snack foods. The 1994 edition of the exchange lists for meal planning are found at the end of this section.

V. **Steps In Planning the Carbohydrate Controlled Diet (example)**

    A. <u>**Establish the calorie level of the diet.**</u> The American Diabetes Association guidelines for nutritional care of individuals with diabetes suggest that 50-60 percent of calories come from carbohydrates. Because the carbohydrate content of the diet is based upon calories, it is necessary to write menus which contain a set daily calorie level. Each might determine the average daily number of calories needed by the majority of diabetic residents who will be receiving the diet. Or, taking the midpoint of calories suggested under the regular diet guidelines would also be appropriate.

    Accepted Calorie Range – Regular Diet   1700-2400
    Suggested Midpoint for the Carbohydrate Controlled Diet 2000

Carbohydrate Controlled Diet

B. **Calculate the daily carbohydrate content in grams.** (Every gram of carbohydrate contains four calories. Fifty to sixty percent of calories from carbohydrate would be acceptable.)

2000 Calories x 55% carbohydrate = 1100 carbohydrate calories per day
1100 carbohydrate calories ÷ 4 calories/gram = <u>275 grams carbohydrate per day</u>

C. **(Plan how the carbohydrates will be distributed throughout the day.)**
There is no single correct way to spread the carbohydrate throughout the day. The goal is to distribute the carbohydrates as evenly as possible but, in general the largest or most popular meals should contain more carbohydrate than lighter meals or snack.

TIP: Because carbohydrate foods in the exchange lists contain an average 15 grams carbohydrate per serving, it is suggested that carbohydrate distribution goals be in multiples of 15 to provide the simplest meal formula.

Example for a facility where meals are approximately the same size:

Breakfast	75 grams carbohydrate (5 carbohydrate servings)
Lunch	75 grams carbohydrate (5 carbohydrate servings)
Dinner	75 grams carbohydrate (5 carbohydrate servings)
Snack	45 grams carbohydrate (3 carbohydrate servings)
Total	270 grams carbohydrate/day*

D. **Other considerations**
1. While the focus of this diet is on total carbohydrates per meal and per day, it is still important to plan menus which are nutritionally balanced and provide at least 2 servings of milk, 2 servings of fruit, 3 servings of vegetables, 6 servings of starch and 5 oz. of protein per day.
2. This diet does not specifically prohibit regular condiments such as regular sugar, regular jelly, regular syrup, etc. However, these foods may be wasted carbohydrates. For example, a single 2 oz. container of regular syrup would "waste" 30 grams of carbohydrate, or two carbohydrate choices, at that meal. This might make it impossible to provide adequate amounts of other carbohydrate foods (e.g. juice and milk) to provide a well-balanced meal.

*Note: The goal for total carbohydrate per day was 275 grams. 270 grams is close enough.

Carbohydrate Controlled Diet

3. This diet allows the diabetic resident to enjoy regular desserts as long as the total carbohydrate within the meal is controlled (see "Other Carbohydrates" exchange list). However, like all well-planned menus, regular dessert should only be included when all nutritional needs have been met and adequate calories remain to allow the regular dessert to be included. Often portions of regular dessert are small so that the menu does not exceed the allowed amount of carbohydrates or calories. At times, a lower sugar, "dietetic" dessert may still be the best choice for a menu. To avoid confusion among staff and residents, it may be wise to try to establish a pattern for incorporating regular desserts - every Sunday and Thursday at the main meal, for example.

VI. EXCHANGE LIST FOR MEAL PLANNING
    See next page.

Carbohydrate Controlled Diet

Traditional Exchange Lists for Meal Planning

Exchange Group	Carbohydrate (g)	Protein (g)	Fat (g)	Calories
Starches	15	3	0-1	80
Fruits	15	-	-	60
Milk				
Skim	12	8	0-1	90
Low Fat	12	8	5	120
Whole	12	8	8	150
Other Carbohydrates	15	varies	varies	-
Vegetables	5	2	-	25
Meat				
Very Lean (VL)	-	7	0-1	35
Lean (L)	-	7	3	55
Medium Fat (MF)	-	7	5	75
High Fat (HF)	-	7	8	100
Fats	-	-	5	45

*Note that the meat and fat exchange groups do not contain carbohydrate.

To simplify meal planning based on carbohydrate content, it is common for starches, fruits, milks and "other carbohydrates" servings to all be averaged to 15 grams of carbohydrate per serving. Foods in any of these groups simply become "carbohydrate foods" and become interchangeable in the diet. For example, on the carbohydrate controlled diet, an 8 ounce glass of skim milk and a medium peach are both calculated to contain 15 grams of carbohydrate. Providing either, would be providing one carbohydrate serving.

Carbohydrate Controlled Diet

Simplified Exchange Lists for Carbohydrate Planning

Exchange Group	Carbohydrate (g)	Protein (g)	Fat (g)	Calories
Starches	15*	3	0-1	80*
Fruits	15*	3	0-1	80*
Milk				
Skim	15*	8	0-1	80*
Low Fat	15	8	5	120
Whole	15	8	8	150
Other Carbohydrates	15	varies	varies	-
Vegetables**	5*	2	-	25
Meat				
Very Lean (VL)	0	7	0-1	35
Lean (L)	0	7	3	55
Medium Fat (MF)	0	7	5	75
High Fat (HF)	0	0	8	100
Fats	0	0	5	45

*It is acceptable to average the carbohydrate and calorie content of the three main "carbohydrate" groups to further simplify meal calculations.

**Because of the small carbohydrate content in vegetables, it is acceptable not to include them in carbohydrate calculations unless three or more exchanges are served together. For example, a chef salad might contain 3 cups of assorted raw vegetables. This would be three vegetable exchanges, 15 grams of carbohydrate, and one serving of carbohydrate.

Other methods of counting carbohydrates, such as nutritional information lists or books, and food labels can also be used in planning the Carbohydrate Controlled Diet. However, there are three benefits of calculating carbohydrate using the exchange lists:

1. Most dietary staff members are already familiar with the exchange lists.
2. Resident preferences can be accommodated more easily. For example, if Mrs. Jones dislikes milk, it is not necessary to rewrite the entire carbohydrate controlled diet for her. Her diet care plan would simply note that the milk in her meals would need to be substituted with another "carbohydrate" serving – such as an extra fruit serving or starch serving – to keep the calculated carbohydrate amounts intact.
3. The same system is used to calculate calorie controlled diabetic diets (see next section), so that the dietary staff does not need to learn two different diabetic diet methods.

Carbohydrate Controlled Diet
Carbohydrate Controlled Meal Plan

(Based upon 55% of calories from carbohydrate or approximately 206 grams) Carbohydrate Distribution 60-65-65-30

Menu	Carbohydrates	Calories

Breakfast

4 oz orange juice (1 fruit)	15	80
¾ cup (1 oz) cold cereal or 4 oz oatmeal (1 starch)	15	80
1 egg, scrambled in PAM (1 MF meat)	0	75
1 piece of toast or 2 - 4" reduced fat pancakes (1 starch)	15	80
1 pat margarine (1 fat)	0	45
1 cup skim milk (1 milk)	15	80
	60	440

Lunch

4 oz orange juice (1 fruit)	15	80
2 oz baked chicken with skin (2 L meat)	0	110
2/3 cup rice, plain (2 starch)	30	160
½ cup carrots plain (1 veg)	5	25
1 pat margarine (1 fat)	0	45
½ cup fresh fruit cup (1 fruit)	15	80
	65	500

Dinner

8 oz vegetable soup	15	80
1 cup tossed salad (1 veg)	5	25
1 packet fat free dressing	0	0
2 slices wheat bread (2 starch)	30	160
½ cup tuna, water-packed (2 VL meat)	0	70
1 tbsp light mayonnaise (1 fat)	0	50
½ cup diet peaches (1 fruit)	15	80
	65	465

Snack

1 cup skim milk (1 milk)	15	80
4 whole wheat crackers (low fat)	15	80
	30	160
DAILY TOTAL	220	1565

Carbohydrate Controlled Diet
Carbohydrate Controlled Meal Plan

(Based upon 55% of calories from carbohydrate or approximately 275 grams) Carbohydrate Distribution 75-75-75-45

One starch exchange equals 15 grams carbohydrate, 3 grams protein 0-1 grams fat and 80 calories.

Menu	Carbohydrates	Calories
Breakfast		
4 oz orange juice (1 fruit)	15	80
¾ cup (1 oz) cold cereal or 4 oz hot cereal (1 starch)	15	80
1 egg, scrambled in PAM (1 MF meat)	0	75
1 piece of toast or 4 - 4" reduced fat pancakes (2 starch)	30	160
2 pats margarine (1 fat)	0	45
1 cup skim milk	<u>15</u>	<u>80</u>
	75	520
Lunch		
1 cup vegetable soup	15	80
2 packet crackers (2 starch)	7.5	40
1 cup tossed salad (1 veg)	trace	25
1 packet light Italian dressing (1 fat)	0	45
2 slices wheat bread (2 starch)	30	160
½ cup tuna, water-packed (2 VL meat)	0	70
1 tbsp light mayonnaise (1 fat)	0	50
½ cup skim milk (1/2 starch)	7.5	40
½ cup chilled peaches (1 starch)	<u>15</u>	<u>80</u>
	75	670
Dinner		
3 oz baked chicken with skin (3 lean meat)	0	165
2/3 cup rice, plain (2 starch)	30	160
6 oz V-8 juice (1 veg)*	15	80
1 cup carrots, plain (2 veg) (*together=1 starch)		
1 roll, small (1 starch)	15	80
1 pat margarine (1 fat)	0	45
½ cup ice cream, vanilla (1 starch, 1 ½ fat)	<u>15</u>	<u>150</u>
	75	670
Snack		
1 cup skim milk (1 starch)	15	80
1 oz angel food cake (1 starch)	15	80
1/2 cup natural applesauce (1 starch)	<u>15</u>	<u>80</u>
	45	240
DAILY TOTAL	270	2020

Carbohydrate Controlled Diet
Carbohydrate Controlled Meal Plan

One starch exchange equals 15 grams carbohydrate, 3 grams protein 0-1 grams fat and 80 calories.

Bread

Bagel	½ (1 oz)
Bread, reduced-calorie	2 slices
Bread, white, whole-wheat	
Pumpernickel or rye	1 slice
Bread sticks, crisp, 4 in long x ½ in	2 (2/3 oz)
English muffin	½
Hot dog or hamburger bun	½ (1 oz)
Pita, 6 in across	1/2
Roll, plain, small	1
Raisin bread, unfrosted	1 slice
Tortilla, corn, 6 in across	1
Waffle, 4 ½ square	
Reduce fat	1

Cereals and Grains

Bran cereals	½ cup
Bulgur	½ cup
Cereals	½ cup
Cereals, unsweetened, ready-to-eat	¾ cup
Cornmeal (dry)	3 tbsp
Couscous	1/3 cup
Flour	3 tbsp
Granola, low fat	¼ cup
Grape nuts	¼ cup
Grits	½ cup
Kasha	1 ½ cup
Millet	¼ cup
Muesli	¼ cup
Oats	½ cup
Pasta	½ cup
Puffed cereal	1 ½ cup
Rice milk	1 ½ cup
Rice, white or brown	1/3 cup
Shredded wheat	1 ½ cup
Sugar-frosted cereal	½ cup
Wheat germ	3 tbsp

Carbohydrate Controlled Diet

One starch exchange equals 15 grams carbohydrate, 3 grams protein 0-1 grams fat and 80 calories.

Starchy Vegetables

Baked beans	1/3 cups
Corn	½ cup
Corn on cob, medium	1 (5 oz)
Mixed vegetables with corn, peas or pasta	1 cup
Plantain	½ cup
Potato (mashed)	1 small (3 oz)
Squash, winter (acorn, butternut)	1 cup
Yam, sweet potato, plain	½ cup

Beans, Peas, and Lentils

Beans and peas (garbanzo, pinto kidney, white, split, black-eyed	½ cup
Lima beans	2/3 cup
Lentils	½ cup
Miscellaneous	3 tbsp

Crackers and Snacks

Animal crackers	8
Graham crackers, 2 ½" Square	3
Matzo	¾ oz
Melba toast	4 slices
Oyster crackers	24
Popcorn (popped, no fat added Or low fat microwave	3 cups
Pretzels	¾ oz
Rice cakes 4 inch across	2
Saltine type crackers	6
Snack chips, fat-free (tortilla, Potato	15-20 (3/4 oz)
Whole-wheat crackers, No fat added	2-5 (3/4 oz)

Carbohydrate Controlled Diet

One starch exchange equals 15 grams carbohydrate, 3 grams protein 0-1 grams fat and 80 calories.

Starchy Foods Prepared with Fat		Common Measurements		
Biscuit, 2 ½ inch across	1	3 tsp	=	1 tbsp
Chow mein noodles	½ cup	4 tbsp	=	¼ cup
Corn bread, 2 in cube	1 (2 oz)	5 1/3 tbsp	=	1/3 cup
Crackers, round butter type	6	4 oz	=	½ cup
Croutons	1 cup	8 oz	=	1 cup
French fried potatoes	16-25 (3 oz)	1 cup	=	½ pint
Granola	¼ cup			
Muffin, small	1 (1 ½ oz)			
Pancake, 4 inch across	2			
Popcorn, microwave	3 cups			
Sandwich cracker, cheese or Peanut butter filling	3			
Stuffing, bread (prepared)	1/3 cup			
Taco, shell, 6 inch square	2			
Waffle, 4 ½ inch square	1			
Whole-wheat crackers, fat added	4-6 (1 oz)			

Starches often swell in cooking so a small amount of uncooked starch will become a much larger amount of cooked food. The following table shows some of the changes.

Food (Starch Group)	Uncooked	Cooked
Oatmeal	3 tbsp	½ cup
Cream of Wheat	2 tbsp	½ cup
Grits	3 tbsp	½ cup
Rice	2 tbsp	1/3 cup
Spaghetti	¼ cup	½ cup
Noodles	1/3 cup	½ cup
Macaroni	¼ cup	½ cup
Dried beans	¼ cup	½ cup
Dried peas	¼ cup	½ cup
Lentils	3 tbsp	½ cup

Carbohydrate Controlled Diet
Fruit Exchanges

One fruit exchange equals 15 grams carbohydrate and 60 calories. The weight includes skin, core, seeds, and rind.

Fruit

Apple, unpeeled, small	1 (4 oz)		
Applesauce, unsweetened	½ cup	Pineapple, canned	½ cup
Apples, dried	4 ring	Plums, small	2 (5 oz)
Apricots, fresh	4 whole (5 ½ oz)	Plums, canned	¼ cup
		Prunes, dried	3
Apricots, dried	8 halves	Raisins	2 tbsp
Apricots, canned	½ cups	Raspberries	1 cup
Banana, small	1 (4 oz)	Strawberries	1 ¼ cup whole berries
Blackberries	¾ cup		
Blueberries	¾ cup	Tangerines, small	2 (8 oz)
Cantaloupe, small	1/3 melon or 1 cup cubes	Watermelon	1 slice or 1 ¼ cup cubes
Cherries, sweet, fresh	12 (3 oz)		
Cherries, sweet, canned	½ cup		
Dates	3	**Fruit Juice**	
Figs, fresh	1 ½ large or 2 medium (3 ½ oz)	Apple juice/cider	½ cup
		Cranberry juice cocktail	1/3 cup
Figs, dried	1 ½ cup	Cranberry juice cocktail, reduced calories	1 cup
Fruit cocktail	½ cup		
Grapefruit, large	½ (11 oz)	Fruit juice blends, 100% juice	1/3 cup
Grapefruit sections, canned	¾ cup		
Grapes, small	17 (3 oz)	Grape juice	1/3 cup
Honeydew melon	1 slice (10 oz) or 1 cup cubes	Grapefruit juice	½ cup
		Orange juice	½ cup
Kiwi	1 (3 ½ oz)	Pineapple juice	½ cup
Mandarin oranges, canned	¾ cup	Prune juice	1/3 cup
Mango, small	½ fruit (5 ½ oz) or 1 cup		
Nectarine, small	1 (5 oz)		
Orange, small	½ fruit (8 oz) or 1 cup cubes		
Papaya	½ fruit (8 oz) or 1 cup cubes		
Peach, medium, fresh	1 (6 oz)		
Peaches, canned	½ cup		
Pear, large, fresh	½ (4 oz)		
Pineapple, fresh	¾ cup		

Carbohydrate Controlled Diet
Milk Exchanges

One milk exchange equals *12 grams carbohydrate and 8 grams protein.

*For ease of menu planning, starches, fruits, and skim milk servings can all be averaged and calculated as 15 grams carbohydrate and 80 calories

Skim and Low fat Milk
(0-3 grams fat per serving)

Reduced Fat
(5 grams fat per serving)

Skim milk	1 cup	2% milk	1 cup
1/2 % skim milk	1 cup	Plain low fat yogurt	¾ cup
1 % milk	1 cup	Sweet acidophilus milk	1 cup
Nonfat or low fat buttermilk	1 cup		
Evaporated skim milk	½ cup		

Whole Milk
(8 grams fat per serving)

Nonfat dry milk	1/3 cup dry	Whole milk	1 cup
Plain nonfat yogurt	1 cup	Evaporated whole milk	½ cup
Nonfat or low fat Fruit-flavored yogurt sweetened with aspartame or with a no nutritive sweetener	1 cup	Goat's milk	1 cup
		Kefir	1 cup

Other Carbohydrates List

You can substitute menu choices from this list for a starch, fruit or milk choice on your meal plan. Some choices will also count as one or more fat choices.

Nutrition Tips

1. These foods can be substituted in your meal plan, even though they contain added sugars or fat. However, they do not contain as many important vitamins and minerals as the choices on the Starch, Fruit or Milk list.

2. When planning to include these foods in your meals, be sure to first include foods from all the lists to provide a balanced meal.

Carbohydrate Controlled Diet
Other Carbohydrates List

3. Because many of these foods are concentrated sources of carbohydrate and fat, the portion sizes are often very small.

4. Many fat-free or reduced fat products made with fat replacers contain carbohydrates. When eaten in large amounts, they may need to be counted. Check labels for carbohydrate content.

5. Use fat-free salad dressings in smaller amounts on the Free Foods lists.

Other Carbohydrates
One exchange equals 15 grams carbohydrate or 1 starch or 1 fruit or 1 milk

Food	Serving Size	Exchanges per Serving
Angel food cake, unfrosted	1/12th cake	2 carbohydrates
Brownie, small unfrosted	2 inch square	1 carbohydrate, 1 fat
Cake, unfrosted	2 inch square	1 carbohydrate, 1 fat
Cake, frosted	2 inch square	2 carbohydrates, 1 fat
Cookie, fat-free	2 small	1 carbohydrate
Cookie or sandwich cookie with cream filling	2 small	1 carbohydrate, 1 fat
Cranberry sauce, jellied	¼ cup	1 ½ carbohydrates
Cupcake, frosted	1 small	2 carbohydrates, 1 fat
Doughnut, plain cake	1 medium (1 ½ oz)	1 ½ carbohydrates, 2 fats
Doughnut, glazed	3 ¾ inch across (2 oz)	2 carbohydrates, 2 fats
Fruit juice bars, frozen, 100% juice	1 bar (3 oz)	1 carbohydrate
Fruit snacks, chewy (pureed fruit concentrate)	1 roll (¾ oz)	1 carbohydrate
Fruit spreads, 100% fruit	1 tbsp	1 carbohydrate
Gelatin, regular	½ cup	1 carbohydrate
Gingersnaps	3	2 carbohydrate
Granola bar	1 bar	1 carbohydrate, 1 fat

Carbohydrate Controlled Diet
Other Carbohydrates

Food	Serving Size	Exchanges per Serving
Honey	1 tbsp	2 carbohydrates
Hummus	1/3 cup	1 carbohydrate, 1 fat
Ice cream	1/3 cup	1 carbohydrate, 1 fat
Ice cream, light	½ cup	1 carbohydrate, 1 fat
Ice cream, fat-free, no sugar added	½ cup	1 carbohydrate
Jam or jelly, regular	1 tbsp	1 carbohydrate
Milk, chocolate, whole	1 cup	2 carbohydrate, 1 fat
Pie, fruit, 2 crusts	1/6 pie	3 carbohydrates, 2 fats
Pie, pumpkin or custard	1/8 pie	2 carbohydrates, 2 fats
Potato chips	12-18 (1 oz)	1 carbohydrate, 2 fat
Pudding, regular (made with low fat milk)	½ cup	2 carbohydrates
Salad dressing, fat-free	¼ cup	2 carbohydrates
Sherbet, sorbet	½ cup	1 carbohydrate
Spaghetti or pasta sauce, canned	1 tbsp	1 carbohydrate, 1 fat
Sugar	1 tbsp	1 carbohydrate
Sweet roll or Danish	1 (2 ½ oz)	2 ½ carbohydrate, 2 fats
Syrup, light	2 tbsp	1 carbohydrate
Syrup, regular	¼ cup	4 carbohydrates
Tortilla chips	6-12 (1 oz)	1 carbohydrate, 2 fats
Vanilla wafers	5	1 carbohydrate, 1 fat
Yogurt, frozen, low fat fat-free	1/3 cup	1 carbohydrate, 0-1 fat
Yogurt, low fat with fruit	1 cup	3 carbohydrates, 0-1 fat

Carbohydrate Controlled Diet
Vegetable Exchange

One vegetable exchange equals 5 grams carbohydrate, 2 grams protein, 0 grams fat and 25 calories.

Artichoke	Okra
Artichoke hearts	Onions
Asparagus	Pea pods
Beans (green, wax, or Italian)	Peppers (all varieties)
Bean sprouts	Radishes
Cabbage	Salad greens (endive, escarole)
Carrots	lettuce, romaine or spinach)
Cauliflower	Sauerkraut
Celery	Spinach
Cucumber	Summer squash
Eggplant green onions or scallions	Tomato
Greens (collard, kale, mustard or turnip)	Tomatoes, canned
Kohlrabi	Tomato sauce
Leeks	Tomato vegetable juice
Mixed vegetables (without corn, peas or pasta)	Turnips

Note: Because the carbohydrate content of this list is so low, 3 servings have to be planned at one time to count as 1 carbohydrate food choice.

1 serving of vegetables is: ½ cup of cooked vegetables, 1 cup of vegetable juice or 1 cup of raw vegetables.

Carbohydrate Controlled Diet
Meat Exchange

Very Lean Meat and Substitutes List
(One exchange equals 0 grams carbohydrate, 7 grams protein, 0-1 grams fat and 35 calories)

One very lean meat exchange is equal to any one of the following items.

Poultry:	Chicken or turkey (white meat, no skin), Cornish hen (no skin)	1 oz
Fish:	Fresh or frozen cod, flounder, haddock, halibut or trout; tuna fresh or canned in water	1 oz
Shellfish:	Clams, crab, lobster, scallops, shrimp, Imitation shellfish	1 oz
Cheese:	With 1 gram or less fat per ounce:	
	Nonfat or low-fat cottage cheese	¼ cup
	Fat-free cheese	1 oz
Other:	Processed sandwich meats with 1 gram or less fat per ounce, such as deli thin, shaved meats, chipped beef, turkey, ham	1 oz
	Egg whites	2
	Egg substitutes, plain	¼ cup
	Hot dogs with 1 gram or less fat per ounce	1 oz
	Kidney (high in cholesterol)	1 oz
	Sausage with 1 gram or less fat per ounce	1 oz
	One very lean meat and one starch exchange is equal to any one of the following items: beans, peas, lentils (cooked)	½ cup

Carbohydrate Controlled Diet
Meat Exchange

Lean Meat and Substitutes List
(One exchange equals 0 grams carbohydrate, 7 grams protein, 3 grams fat and 55 calories)

One lean meat exchange is equal to any one of the following items.

Beef:	USDA Select or Choice grades of lean beef trimmed of fat, such as round, sirloin and flank steak; tenderloin, roast (rib, chuck or rump); steak (T-bone, porterhouse or cubed), ground round	1 oz
Pork:	Lean pork, such as fresh ham; canned, cured or Boiled ham; Canadian bacon; tenderloin, center Loin chop	1 oz
Lamb:	Roast, chop, leg	1 oz
Veal:	Lean chop, roast	1 oz
Poultry:	Chicken, turkey (dark meat, no skin), chicken (white meat, with skin), domestic duck or goose (well-drained of fat no skin)	1 oz
Fish:	Herring (uncreamed or smoked)	1 oz
	Oysters	6 medium
	Salmon (fresh or canned), catfish	1 oz
	Sardines (canned)	2 medium
	Tuna (canned in oil, drained)	1 oz
Game:	Goose (no skin), rabbit	1 oz
Cheese:	4.5% fat cottage cheese	¼ cup
	Grated Parmesan	2 tbsp
	Cheeses with 3 grams or less fat per ounce	1 oz
Other:	Hot dogs with 3 grams or less fat per ounce	1 ½ oz
	Processed sandwich meat with 3 grams or less fat per ounce, such as turkey pastrami or kielbasa	1 oz
	Liver, heart (high in cholesterol)	1 oz

Carbohydrate Controlled Diet
Meat Exchanges

Medium Fat Meat and Substitutes List
(One exchange equals 0 grams carbohydrate, 7 grams protein, 5 grams fat and 75 calories)

One medium fat meat exchange is equal to any one of the following items.

Beef:	Most beef products fall into this category; ground beef, meatloaf, corned beef, short ribs, prime grades of meat trimmed of fat, such as prime rib	1 oz
Pork:	Top loin, chop, Boston butt cutlet	1 oz
Lamb:	Rib roast, ground	1 oz
Veal:	Cutlet (ground or cubed, unbreaded)	1 oz
Poultry:	Chicken (dark meat, with skin), ground turkey or ground chicken, fried chicken (with skin)	1 oz
Fish:	Any fried fish product	1 oz
Cheese:	With 5 grams or less fat per ounce:	
	Feta	1 oz
	Mozzarella	1 oz
	Ricotta	2 oz (1/4 cup)
Other:	Egg (high in cholesterol, limit 3 per week)	1
	Sausage with 5 grams or less fat per ounce	1
	Soy milk	1 cup
	Tempeh	¼ cup
	Tofu	4 oz or ½ cup

Carbohydrate Controlled Diet
Meat Exchanges

High Fat Meat and Substitutes List
(One exchange equals 0 grams carbohydrate, 7 grams protein, 8 grams fat and 100 calories)

Remember these items are high in saturated fat, cholesterol and calories and may raise blood cholesterol levels if eaten on a regular basis.

One high fat meat exchange is equal to any of the following items.

Pork:	Spare ribs, ground pork, pork sausage	1 oz
Cheese:	All regular cheeses, such as: American, Cheddar, Monterey Jack or Swiss	1 oz
Other:	Processed sandwich meats with 8 grams or less fat per ounce, such as bologna, pimento loaf and salami	1 oz
	Sausage, such as bratwurst, Italian, or Knockwurst, Polish, smoked	1 oz
	Hot dog (turkey or chicken)	1 (10/lb)
	Bacon	3 slices (10 slices/lb)

One high fat meat exchange plus one fat exchange is equal to one of the following items:

Hot dog (beef, pork or combination)   1 (10/lb)

One high fat meat exchange plus two fat exchanges is equal to the following item:

Peanut butter (contains unsaturated fat)   2 tbsp

Carbohydrate Controlled Diet
Meat Exchanges

Monounsaturated Fats List
(One fat exchange equals 5 grams fat and 45 calories)

Avocado:	Medium	1/8 (1 oz)
Oil:	Canola, olive or peanut	1 tsp
Olives:	Ripe (black)	8 large
	Green, stuffed	10 large
Nuts:	Cashews, almonds	6 nuts
	Mixed (50% peanuts)	6 nuts
	Peanuts	10 nuts
	Pecans	4 halves
	Peanut butter, smooth or crunch	2 tsp
	Sesame seeds	1 tbsp
	Tahini paste	2 tsp

Polyunsaturated Fats list
(One fat exchange equals 5 grams fat and 45 calories)

Margarine:	Stick, tub or squeeze	1 tsp
	Lower fat (30% to 50% vegetable oil)	1 tsp
Nuts:	Walnuts, English	4 halves
Oil:	Corn, Safflower or Soybean	1 tsp
Salad dressing:	Regular	1 tbsp
	Reduced fat	2 tbsp
	Miracle Whip® salad dressing	
	Regular	2 tsp
	Reduced fat	1 tbsp
Seeds:	Pumpkin, sunflower	1 tbsp

Carbohydrate Controlled Diet
Meat Exchanges

Saturated Fats List
(One fat exchange equals 5 grams fat and 45 calories)

Bacon:	Cooked	1 slice (20 slices/lb)
Butter:	Stick	1 tsp
	Whipped	2 tsp
	Reduced fat	1 tbsp
Chitterlings:	Boiled	2 tbsp (1/2 oz)
Coconut:	Sweetened, shredded	2 tbsp
Cream:	Half and half	2 tbsp
Cream cheese:	Regular	1 tbsp (1/2 oz)
	Reduced fat	2 tbsp
Shortening or lard:		1 tsp
Sour cream:	Regular	2 tbsp
	Reduced fat	3 tbsp

Carbohydrate Controlled Diet
Free Foods

A free food is any food or drink that contains less than 20 calories or less than 5 grams of carbohydrate per serving. Foods with a serving size listed should be limited to three servings per day. Be sure to spread them out throughout the day.

Fat free or Reduced fat Foods

Food	Serving
Cream cheese, fat free	1 tbsp
Creamers, non dairy, liquid	1 tbsp
Creamers, non dairy, powder	2 tsp
Mayonnaise, fat free	1 tbsp
Mayonnaise, reduced fat	1 tsp
Margarine, fat free	4 tbsp
Margarine, reduced fat	1 tsp
Miracle Whip®, non fat	1 tbsp
Miracle Whip®, reduced fat	1 tsp
Nonstick cooking spray	-
Salad dressing, fat free	1 tbsp
Salad dressing, fat free, Italian	2 tbsp
Salsa	¼ cup
Sour cream, fat free, reduced fat	1 tbsp
Whipped topping, regular or light	2 tbsp

Carbohydrate Controlled Diet
Free Foods

Sugar free or low sugar foods

Candy, hard, sugar free	1 tbsp
Gelatin dessert, sugar free	-
Gelatin, unflavored	-
Gum, sugar free	-
Jam or jelly, low sugar or light	2 tsp
Sugar substitutes*	
Syrup, sugar free	2 tbsp

* Sugar substitutes, alternatives or replacements that are approved by the Food and Drug Administration (FDA) are safe to use. Common brand names include:

Equal®, (aspartame)
Sprinkle Sweet® (saccharin)
Sweet One® (acesulfame K)
Sweet-10® (saccharin)
Sugar Twin® (saccharin)
Sweet'n Low® (saccharin)
Splenda® (sucralose)

Carbohydrate Controlled Diet
Free Foods

Drinks

Bouillon, Broth, consommé	-
Bouillon or broth, low-sodium	-
Carbonated or mineral water	-
Club soda	-
Cocoa powder, unsweetened	1 tbsp
Coffee	-
Diet soft drinks, sugar free	-
Drink mixes, sugar free	-
Tea, Tonic water, sugar free	-

Carbohydrate Controlled Diet
Free Foods

Condiments

Catsup	1 tbsp
Horseradish	1 tsp
Lemon juice	-
Mustard	-
Pickles, dill	1 ½ large
Soy Sauce, regular or light	1 tbsp
Taco sauce	1 tbsp
Vinegar	-

Seasonings

Flavoring extract	-
Garlic	-
Herbs, fresh or dried	-
Pimiento	-
Spices	-
Tabasco® or hot pepper sauce	-
Wine, used in cooking	-
Worchester sauce	-

Carbohydrate Controlled Diet
Combination Foods List

Food Entrees	Serving Size	Exchanges per Serving
Tuna noodle casserole, lasagna, spaghetti with meatballs, chili with beans or macaroni and cheese	1 cup (8 oz)	2 carbohydrates, 2 medium fat meats
Chow mein (without noodles or rice)	2 cups (16 oz)	1 carbohydrate, 2 lean meats
Pizza, cheese, thin crust	¼ of 10 in (5 oz)	2 carbohydrates, 2 medium fat meats, 2 fats
Pizza, meat topping, Thin crust	¼ of 10 in (5 oz)	2 carbohydrates, 2 medium fat meats, 2 fats
Pot pie	1 (7 oz)	2 carbohydrates, 1 medium fat meats, 4 fats
Frozen Entrees		
Salisbury steak with gravy	1 (11 oz)	2 carbohydrates, 3 medium fat meats, 3-4 fats
Turkey with gravy, mashed potatoes, and dressing	1 (11 oz)	1 carbohydrate, 1 fat 2 carbohydrates
Entree with less than 300 Calories	1 (8 oz)	2 carbohydrates, 3 lean meats

Carbohydrate Controlled Diet
Combination Foods List

Food Entrees	Serving Size	Exchanges per Serving
Soup		
Bean	1 cup	1 carbohydrates, 1 very lean meat
Cream Soup (made with water)	1 cup (8 oz)	1 carbohydrate, 1 fat
Split pea (made with water)	½ cup (4 oz)	1 carbohydrate
Tomato (made with water)	1 cup (8 oz)	1 carbohydrate
Vegetable beef, chicken noodle or other broth-type	1 cup (8 oz)	1 carbohydrate

Carbohydrate Controlled Diet

Fast Food Entrees	Serving Size	Exchanges per Serving
Burritos with beef	2	4 carbohydrates, 2 medium fat meats, 2 fats
Chicken nuggets	6	1 carbohydrate, 2 medium fat meats, 1 fat
Chicken breast and wing, breaded and fried	1 each	1 carbohydrate, 4 medium fat meats, 2 fats
Fish sandwich with tartar sauce	1	3 carbohydrate, 1 medium fat meat, 3 fats
French fries, thin	20-25	2 carbohydrates, 2 fats
Hamburger, regular	1	2 carbohydrates, 2 medium fat meat
Hamburger, large	1	2 carbohydrates, 3 medium fat meats, 1 fat
Hot dog with bun	1	1 carbohydrate, 1 high fat meat, 1 fat
Individual pan pizza	1	5 carbohydrates, 3 medium fat meats, 3 fats
Soft serve cone	1 medium	2 carbohydrates, 1 fat
Submarine sandwich	1 sub (6 in)	3 carbohydrates, 1 vegetable, 2 medium fat meats, 1 fat
Taco, hard shell	1 (6 oz)	2 carbohydrates, 2 medium fat meats, 2 fats
Taco, soft shell with meat	1 (3 oz)	1 carbohydrate, 1 medium fat meat, 1 fat

Calorie Restricted Diet (Low Calorie)

I. **Description**
The low calorie diet is indicated when reduction in weight is desirable and resident agrees. The diet follows the pattern for the regular diet with modification made in total calorie content. It provides a range of 1200-1800 calories.

*See the Carbohydrate Controlled Diet Plan for "Free Foods" and "Foods for Occasional Use" for additional suggestions

II. **Approximate Composition**
Calories   1200-1800 based on individual calculated needs and preferences
Protein   60-75 grams

III. **Adequacy**
This diet includes the basic food groups in adequate amounts but fats and carbohydrates are limited to reduce total calories below normal requirements.

Limited Concentrated Sweets (LCS) Diet

I. Description

This diet closely resembles the regular diet, restricting only those foods which are high in sugar or other concentrated sweets. It can be used for any diabetic patient whose weight and blood sugar levels are under control. It does not require adherence to a strict meal pattern nor does it necessarily restrict calories.

II. Approximate Composition

Calories   1600-2000
Protein   60-75 grams

III. Adequacy

This diet contains all nutrients necessary to provide and maintain adequate nutrition based on the Dietary Guidelines for Americans 2010.

FOOD GROUPS	FOODS INCLUDED	FOODS EXCLUDED
Milk	All types	Chocolate milk, sweetened condensed milk
Meat and equivalent	All types	Glazed, honey coated meats or prepared with sugar or syrup
Fruits	All types	Fruit canned or frozen in syrup, sugar or syrup sweetened juices; candied fruit
Vegetables	All types	Candied vegetables

Limited Concentrated Sweets (LCS) Diet

FOOD GROUPS	FOODS INCLUDED	FOODS EXCLUDED
Soups	All types	Fruit soups made with sugar
Breads, Cereal & Grains	All types	Danish rolls, sweet rolls, glazed doughnuts, sugary cereals
Fats	All types	None
Desserts*	Any made with foods allowed; small serving frosted cake(1" x 2"), ice cream, plain cakes and cookies (no icing), ice milk sherbet, sweetened limited to 3 times per week.	Regular potion size of; cake with frosting, cookies with icing, pudding, gelatin, other dessert items
Beverages	All types without added sugar	Beverages sweetened with sugar
Miscellaneous	Sugar substitutes; dietetic and all-fruit jam, jelly, preserves; low calorie diet syrup cocoa powder chocolate flavoring herbs, spices, flavorings salt, catsup, vinegar, pickles, mustard, Worcestershire sauce, soy sauce	Sugar, regular jam, jelly, preserves, syrup, honey, molasses

*See the Carbohydrate Controlled Diet for the "Free Foods" and "Foods for Occasional Use"

Sample Menu Plan
Breakfast

Fruit or juice	Orange juice	4 ounces
Cereal	Oatmeal	½ cup
Meat or equivalent	Scramble eggs	1
Bread	Toast, whole wheat	1 slice
Fat	Soft margarine	1 packet
Milk	2% milk	8 ounces
Beverage	of choice	6-8 ounces
Miscellaneous	Jelly, diet	1 packet
	Sugar substitute	2 packets
	Creamer	as desired
	Salt, Pepper	1 packet each

Lunch or Supper

Meat or equivalent	Tuna salad	½ cup
Vegetable	Vegetable soup	6 ounces
Salad	Tossed salad	1 cup
Fat	Italian dressing	1 ounce
Fat	Mayonnaise	1 tablespoon
Bread	Whole wheat bread	2 slices
Dessert	Chilled peaches	½ cup
Milk	2% milk	8 ounces
Beverage	of choice	6-8 ounces
Miscellaneous	Sugar substitute	1-2 packets
	Creamer	as desired
	Salt, Pepper	1 packet each

Dinner

Meat or equivalent	Baked chicken breast (without skin)	3 ounces (cooked) (½ breast)
Potato or equivalent	Mashed potato/gravy	½ cup/1 ounce
Fat	Soft margarine	1 teaspoon
Milk	2% milk	8 ounces
Vegetable	Seasoned carrots	½ cup
Salad	Mixed fruit salad	½ cup
Bread	Dinner roll, whole wheat	1
Dessert	Diet vanilla ice cream	½ cup
Beverage	of choice	6-8 ounces
Miscellaneous	Sugar substitute	1-2 packets
	Creamer	as desired
	Salt, Pepper	1 packet each

Evening Nourishment

	Juice	4 ounces
	Graham crackers	3 squares

Diabetic Diet (Calculated)

SUGGESTED MEAL PLANS

Suggested plans for diabetic caloric controlled diets are based on the use of medium fat meat and skim milk exchanges.

	CALORIES		
	1200	1500	1800
Breakfast			
Milk	1	1	1
Vegetable	-	-	-
Fruit	1	1	1
Bread	1	2	2
Meat	1	1	1
Fat	1	1	1
Lunch			
Milk	-	-	-
Vegetable	1	1	1
Fruit	1	2	2
Bread	1	2	3
Meat	2	2	2
Fat	0	1	1
Dinner			
Milk	-	-	1
Vegetable	1	1	1
Fruit	2	2	2
Bread	1	2	2
Meat	2	2	2
Fat	0	1	1
Evening Nourishment			
Milk	1	1	1
Bread	1	1	1
Total exchanges per day			
Milk	2	2	3
Vegetable	2	2	2
Fruit	4	5	5
Bread	4	7	8
Meat	5	5	5
Fat	2	3	5

Lactose Reduced Diet

I. **Description**

The lactose reduced diet is used for residents who can consume a moderate amount of lactose (milk sugar) in their daily diets without symptoms of lactose intolerance such as gastrointestinal cramping, gas and diarrhea. Residents who exhibit such symptoms after consuming even a small amount of lactose, should follow a strict regimen that eliminates all sources of lactose.

When planning the daily menu, the list of Lactose Content of Foods which follows should be consulted to avoid exceeding the amount of lactose. The meals should also be planned to meet the individual tolerance of each resident.

Those residents who can tolerate milk treated with lactase, the enzyme which reduces lactose to the monosaccharides glucose and galactose may use it as freely as tolerated. The enzyme can be purchased and added to the milk before use (read the label for directions). The enzyme in tablet form can be taken orally immediately before consuming an offending food. Milk already treated with the enzyme and ready for consumption is available commercially. Additionally, consuming milk with a meal improves lactose tolerance.

II. **Approximate Composition**

Calories 1600-2000
Protein 60-75 grams
Lactose as tolerated

Calcium and Vitamin D supplements may be indicated if milk products are very restricted.

III. **Adequacy**

Based on the Dietary Guidelines for Americans 2010. This diet is inadequate in calcium, riboflavin and vitamin D.

Lactose Reduced Diet
Lactose Content of Food

Foods		Grams of Lactose
Milk	Whole, skim, buttermilk or chocolate	9-13
	Sweetened condensed (1 cup)	35
Cream	Light, heavy, sour (2 tablespoons)	1-2
Yogurt	8 ounces	10-15
Butter	2 pats (10 gm)	.1
Margarine	-	0
Ice cream	Ice milk (1 cup)	9-10
Sherbet	Orange (1 cup)	4
Cheese	1 ounce	
	Brick, Feta, Liederkranz, Muenster Provolone, Romano, Roquefort	0
	Bleu, Brie, Cheddar, Colby, Limburger	.7
	Camembert, Mozzarella	.1
	Cottage, ½ cup	
	creamed	2.5-3
	uncreamed	3.5-4
	Cream	.8
	Edam, Neufchatel	.3
	Gouda	.3-.6
	Parmesan	.9
	Primost	12.2
	Ricotta	.4-1
	Swiss	1.7
	Pasteurized processed, American, Swiss, Pimento	.4-1.7

*Most commercially prepared nutritional supplements and tube feeding formulas are lactose free. Read labels to verify the nutritional content of the products being used.

Kosher Diet

I. Description

The Kosher diet is based on the Biblical rules for food (dietary laws) for the Jewish religion. It may be best to consult a Rabbi in your area for specific questions related to the diet as rules can be very complex. For those wishing a kosher diet, one should interview the individual or a family member to determine the extent of their observance to the diet. Some may accept foods coming from a non-kosher kitchen, while others may not. The Kosher diet may also be an acceptable diet for those practicing the Muslim religion.

The Kosher Diet rules pertain mainly to the selection, slaughter and preparation of meats. All animals and fowl must be inspected for disease and must be slaughtered according to specific rules. Blood is forbidden for consumption. The koshering process removes all blood before cooking. This is achieved by soaking the meat in water, salting it thoroughly, draining and washing it three times to remove the salt. Only the forequarter of the quadrupeds with cloven hooves that chew cud are allowed (i.e. bison, cattle, deer, goats, sheep). The hindquarter of quadrupeds is not allowed except when the hip sinew of the thigh vein is removed. In order to meet the rules for a Kosher Diet, any meat must come from a kosher butcher.

Chicken, duck, goose, pheasant and turkey are allowed. Eggs may be eaten, however, eggs with any blood in the yolk are not allowed. Fish with fins and scales, but should not be consumed with meat. Shellfish, catfish, squid and eel are not allowed.

Milk and milk products may not be consumed with meat. Separate dishes, glasses and utensils must be used for milk verses meat meals. A facility that does not have a kosher kitchen may choose to use disposables for all dairy meals. Milk and or milk products may be consumed immediately before a meat meal, but not with a meat meal. The individual must wait 6 hours after eating meat before milk can be consumed. Eggs may be eaten with milk or meat. Foods that are considered neutral (pareve or "parve") may be eaten with any meal: fruits, vegetables, grains, eggs, non-dairy beverages.

Kosher kitchen keep two completely separate kitchens to separate equipment, dishes and silverware (one for meat and one for milk meals). Saturday is the Sabbath day (day of rest) and no food may be cooked on the Sabbath. All foods to be eaten on the Sabbath must be cooked the day before and held in the oven or served cold. Friday evening meal is usually large and includes brisket and chicken.

All foods must be prepared under kosher standards and have the appropriate hechsher (symbol for kosher). Fresh fruits and vegetables must be free of any insects. Any prepared food mixtures must be made under kosher standards.

Kosher certified items are fairly readily available in the US. Pre-cooked frozen kosher meals are available, but when reheated in a non-kosher oven they must be covered with two layers of foil, or in a non-kosher microwave, by double wrapping the food.

Kosher Diets follow the biblical rules for food for the Jewish Religion which pertain mainly to the selection, slaughter and preparation of meals. Only kosher meats, fish and poultry are allowed. All foods except of fresh fruits and vegetables must be produced under Kosher Standards and have appropriate hechsher (symbol for kosher). These guidelines are intended for use with adults. To meet 100% of the US RDA/AI for the majority of individuals as defined by the National Research Council, provide adequate nutrients by following these daily guidelines to plan three balanced meals and up to three snacks.

II. Approximate Composition

Calories 1800-2200
Protein 60-77 grams

III. Adequacy

This diet contains all nutrients necessary to provide and maintain adequate Nutrition based on the Dietary Guidelines for Americans 2010

Food Item	Amount Each Day
Protein Foods (fish seafood, lean meat, poultry eggs, dried beans/peas/lentils, soy products, nuts, etc.) Fish eggs and peanut butter are pareve. If they are made as part of the meat meal they are considered "meat" and cannot be consumed with milk. If they are prepared as part of the dairy meal they can be consumed with dairy. Do not consume with milk.	5-6 oz or equivalent Encourage 8 oz of cooked seafood per week **NOTE: Must wait 6 hours after eating meat before consuming milk**
Dairy (fortified with vitamins A and D) Do not consume with meat – must wait 6 hours after eating meat before consuming milk.	3 cups or equivalent: 1 cup is equal to 1 cup of liquid milk or yogurt, 1 ½ oz natural cheese or 2 oz processed cheese
Fruits (include a variety) with more whole fruit than juice as appropriate	≥ 1 ½ cups or equivalent : ½ cup equals ½ cup canned, juice or 1 piece fresh
Vegetables (include more dark green and leafy, red/orange vegetables) dry beans/peas/lentils	≥ 2 cups or equivalent: ½ cup equals ½ cup cooked/canned, juice or 1 cup raw
Grains (include as much whole grain/enriched as possible) at least half grains should be whole	≥ 6 oz equivalent: 1 oz equals 1 slice bread, ½ bun or bagel, 1 cup cold cereal, ½ cup hot cereal, ½ cup cooked rice or pasta
Fluids (especially water)	≥ 8 (8 oz) glasses of fluid daily. ≥ 1500 Ml unless contraindicated
Solid Fats and Added Sugars (SoFAS) Avoid added fats, saturated fats, trans fats & sugars. Most fat should come from healthy oils	Use in limited quantities to round out the menu for a pleasing appearance, and satisfying meals. Alcohol in moderation and appropriate

Follow menus & recipes approved by RD, LDN

Kosher Symbols

O or O – Signifies that the product is considered kosher. Additional symbols that may be used with the O or O : D - Signifies that the product is acceptable with dairy meals (it has dairy ingredients) DE – Signifies that the product is acceptable with milk meals (it may also be processed on equipment that also processes dairy ingredients	M – Signifies that the product is acceptable with meat/poultry meals (it contains meat/poultry or is processed on equipment that also processes meat/poultry. P - Signifies that the product is kosher for Passover, but may not be Pareve (non-milk or meat) Kochsher symbol for Kosher

There are many kosher symbols which are specific to the certifying agency where the food is processed.

Jewish Holidays

Rosh Hashanah is the Jewish New Years which is celebrated in September.
Yom Kippur is the Day of Atonement. It occurs 10 days after Rosh Hashanah. Yom Kippur is a day of fasting; no food or beverages of any kind may be consumed from sundown the evening before Yom Kippur until sundown on the day of Yom Kippur. (The two exceptions are for people who are ill and pregnant women)
Passover occurs in the spring and lasts for eight days. During this time leavened bread and cakes is not allowed. Instead, Matzah, an unleavened bread is served. All cake and baked goods are made from ground Matzah or potato starch, and leavened only with whipped egg whites. Iodized salt is not allowed in the traditional Passover Matzah. Any grain or product made from barley, corn, rice, rye or wheat is restricted during Passover, as are dried beans, peas, and soybeans. The kitchen and all equipment are thoroughly cleaned to remove traces of leavened bread or "chometz". The usual pans, dishes, plates, and silverware cannot be used for Passover food. Different pans, dishes, cups and silverware are used especially for, and only for Passover. All foods, except fresh fruits and vegetables (including beverages), must be certified "kosher for Passover".
Purim is a spring celebration. A traditional triangle shaped, filled cookie called Hamentashen is served.
Succot is a fall harvest holiday.
Chanukah is the Festival of Lights which is celebrated for 8 days in mid winter. Foods traditionally served are fried in oil i.e., latkes (potato pancakes) and sufganiot (doughnuts).

Foods Allowed	Foods to Avoid
Protein Foods (Low fat as appropriate) Kosher beef, lamb, mutton, veal, goat, or deer meat. Kosher chicken, duck, goose, pheasant or turkey. Kosher Frankfurters, deli meats. Fish with fins and scales: bluefish, cod, haddock hake, halibut, salmon, scrod, swordfish, tuna. Eggs from domestic fowl	Any non-kosher meat or poultry. Pork (bacon, ham, Canadian bacon, sausage) Rabbit Regular Frankfurters, deli meat. Shellfish (clams, crab, lobster, mussels, oysters, shrimp), eel, frog, octopus, shark, (**Note:** Fish should not be consumed with meat. Milk may be consumed immediately *before* a meat meal but *not with* a meat meal. One must wait 6 hours after consuming meat to drink milk.
Dairy (Low fat as appropriate) Kosher cheese (May not be served with meat) and other milk products	All dairy when meat is served. Non-kosher cheese, cheese served with meat. *Note:* Meat may not be served with milk and milk products. Milk may be consumed immediately before a meat meal but not with a meat meal. One must wait 6 hours after consuming meat to drink milk.
Fruits All canned and frozen fruits identified as Kosher	Any canned or frozen fruits which are not identified as Kosher.
Vegetables (Low fat as appropriate) All fresh Kosher canned or frozen.	Non-kosher vegetable products (canned or frozen) No sauces containing dairy are allowed when meat is served.
Grains (Low fat as appropriate) Bakery items prepared under kosher standards. (If it contains dairy, may not be eaten with meat).	Any bakery items that are not prepared by kosher standards (or containing animal fat such as lard).
Fluids All except those listed under foods to avoid	Non-kosher canned or frozen vegetable juices
Solid Fats and Added Sugars (SoFAS), Alcohol and Miscellaneous Kosher alcohol, beer or wine. Beverages made from crystal powders, carbonated beverages, coffee, tea. Any prepared food mixtures prepared under kosher standards (desserts, soups, etc) Pudding, ice cream or sherbet with dairy meals only. Kosher candy, chocolate, jam, jelly, honey, pepper, salt, sugar, sugar substitutes.	Animal fats (bacon grease or lard) Dark Beer Non-kosher desserts, soups Gelatin or products made with gelatin, unless identified as Kosher by the hechsher (symbol for Kosher) Marshmallows Non-kosher candy, grape jam, jelly. Beverages that are not identified as Kosher.

Kosher Diet

Sample Daily Meal Plan for a Well Balanced Diet

Breakfast	Lunch	Dinner
½ c Orange Juice ½ c Oatmeal ¼ c Scrambled Eggs 1 slice Whole Wheat Toast 1 tbsp Jelly or Fruit Spread 1 tsp Margarine* 1 c Low Fat Milk and /or Yogurt Condiments as Desired+ Beverage of Choice	3 oz Kosher Roast Beef ½ c Seasoned Rice ½ c Seasoned Peas w/Mushrooms 1 c. Green Salad Dressing 1 Whole Wheat Roll ½ c Fruit Sorbet with ¼ cup Strawberries **No Milk** Condiments as Desired+ Beverage of Choice	6 oz Vegetable Soup 2 oz Baked Fish ½ c Mashed Potato ½ c Green Beans 1 Slice Bread 1 Baked Apple 1 c Low Fat Milk **(6 hours later than lunch)** Condiments as Desired+ Beverage of Choice
P.M. Snack		
2 Kosher Cookies 1 c Milk		

Bold/ italicized items indicate differences from a Regular Diet menu
*Low in Trans fats
+May include pepper or other spices, sugars, sugar substitute, salt, coffee creamer, etc. based on nutrition goals

Recommended Nutritional Composition	
Calories 1800 - 2200	**Fluids** based on individual needs
Carbohydrates 45 – 65% of Calories	**Sodium** 2300 mg (higher with processed/convenience foods and added salt)
Protein 10 – 35% of Calories	**Calcium** ≥ 1000 – 1200 mg **Vitamin D** 600 – 800 IU
Fat 20 – 35% of Calories <10% from sat. fat <300 mg cholesterol	**Vitamin C** 90 mg
Nutrients may vary day to day, but should average to the above estimates	

Enteral Nutrition

I. **Description**

Feeding tubes may be used to deliver enteral formulas to residents who are unable to meet nutritional requirements with oral intake and who have a functioning gastrointestinal tract. A tube may be passed through the nasal passage to the stomach (nasogastric) or on into the small intestine (nasoduodenal or nasojejunostomy). Or a tube may be placed through a stoma (opening) in the abdomen, directly into the stomach (gastrostomy) or small intestine (jejunostomy). Careful consideration should be taken to ensure the residents wishes are honored prior to inserting a feeding tube.

A variety of formulas are available to meet the specific needs of each resident. When choosing a formula, it is important to take into account the resident's specific nutritional needs, clinical condition, and the route of administration. Standard enteral formulas provide 1-1.2 Kcal/ml. Concentrated solutions (1.5-2.0 kcal/ml) are appropriate for residents on a fluid restriction or who have high caloric needs. Semi-elemental formulas, containing protein in a mixture of elemental amino acids and dipeptides are recommended for residents who have malabsorption disorders or are unable to tolerate other formulas. Fiber-containing formulas are used to assist with bowel regulation.

Periodically flushing the tubing helps to maintain its patency. Fluids recommended for flushing include water, normal saline and half-normal saline. Fluids such as cola beverages and cranberry juice are not recommended as rinsing agents; the dried residues can further narrow the lumen of the tube and contribute to clogging.

All feedings must be monitored for tolerance and the volume of enteral formula administered should be recorded. The enteral feeding schedule should take into account planned downtime to ensure the total daily volume is delivered.

The physician is responsible for ordering enteral access placement and the tube feeding regimen. The order should include:

1. Name of the product
2. Total daily volume to be delivered
3. Route of administration
4. Method of administration
5. Strength of solution, and if not full-strength the order must include a planned schedule to increase to full strength
6. Intermittent Feeding: number of feedings per day with amount (in ml) of formula for each feeding.

Enteral Nutrition

7. Continuous Feedings: hourly rate (in ml) of formula and the number of hours per day, start time and end time for the feeding
8. Flushes: volume and number of times the tubing is to be flushed, and the content of the flushes
9. Amount of water to be used with medications
10. Total calories to be delivered per day

II. Composition

The nutritional content of the tube feeding will depend upon the amount and type of formula used.

III. Adequacy

A variety of commercial tube feeding formulas are available to meet specific needs of each resident. Care should be taken to note the volume specified by the manufacturer to achieve 100 percent of the Recommended Dietary Allowances for vitamins and minerals. If a lesser volume is to be delivered, a vitamin/mineral supplement (preferably liquid) should be given daily. If the formula falls short of macronutrient requirements (e.g. protein, carbohydrate or fat), modular products are available that can be added to the formula to meet the estimated daily needs.

A thorough nutritional assessment of the individual should be conducted prior to determining the desired formula, rate and strength. In addition to determining daily protein, calorie and fluid needs, the assessment should consider specific micronutrient needs that may be higher for that individual (e.g. iron, calcium, etc.). Calculation of the final content of the tube feeding should include a free-water calculation, and additional flushes ordered to meet the individual's fluid needs.

Tube feeding products are classified in a number different ways including: isotonic, elemental, semi-elemental and intact protein containing formulas, high calorie, high protein, fiber added, specialty formulas, etc. Manufacturers provide product handbooks for complete information on each formula. Information on many formulas is also available online.

Enteral Nutrition

IV. Methods of Administration

Enteral feedings may be given in a variety of ways.

Continuous Feeding
Continuous feedings are administered at a constant rate over a 16-24 hour period using a gravity flow set or a feeding pump to control the flow of the formula. A feeding pump should be used for feeding into the duodenum or jejunum as the small bowel is unable to tolerate larger volumes and sudden rate changes. Continuous feeding is associated with lower residual volumes and reduced risk of aspiration.

Cyclic Feeding
Cyclic feedings are delivered continuously, but at an increased rate over 8-16 hours, often overnight, using a pump. This method favors increased oral intake during the day for individuals receiving a tube feeding as a supplemental nutrient source. It also provides greater mobility to the individual during the day and is a good method to use when transitioning residents from enteral feeding to an oral diet.

Intermittent Feedings
Intermittent feedings can be given at specific intervals during the day, often patterned after a normal meal schedule, and are given by gravity drip or feeding pump over 30-120 minute period. This method is useful for residents in rehabilitation.

Bolus Feedings
Bolus feedings are usually given in less than 15 minutes via a syringe, or feeding bag. The feeding should be initiated as no more than 120 mL of isotonic formula every 4 hours, advancing by 60 ml every 8-1 hours as tolerated. Bolus feedings should not exceed 400-500 mL per feeding.

/

Parenteral Nutrition

Parenteral nutrition (PN) is a means of providing intravenous protein, carbohydrate, fat, vitamins, and mineral to those who are unable to be adequately fed via the gastrointestinal (GI) tract.

When PN provides for all of the macronutrient needs of the resident, it is referred to as total parenteral nutrition (TPN) and must be provided via a central venous catheter or a peripherally inserted central catheter (PICC). Indications for TPN include: GI fistulas, severe pancreatitis, severe catabolism/malnutrition with inability to feed less than or equal to 5 days, intractable vomiting, short bowel syndrome, inflammatory bowel disease with need for bowel rest, and major surgery with inability to feed within 7-10 days post-surgery.

TPN should only be used when other means of nutrition support are unavailable, as it presents a significant risk to the patient. Common complications include: hyperglycemia, catheter-related sepsis, and electrolyte imbalances.

When PN is provided via a peripheral vein, it is referred to as peripheral parenternal nutrition (PPN). The primary purpose of PPN is to provide sufficient macronutrients to meet the needs of glycolysis, and spare protein stores. It is generally used for residents with a short-term (less than or equal to 5 days) inability to utilize the GI tract. It is not adequate for residents with severe malnutrition.

Nutrient content of PN components

Lipid:
20% lipid = 2 kcal/ml
10% lipid = 1.1 kcal/ml

Carbohydrate:
D50=50% dextrose
D25=25% dextrose, etc.
1 gm dextrose = 3.4 Kcal

Protein:
Protein=% (amino acid) aa s
1 gm protein = 4 Kcal

Calculation of TPN Solutions

The TPN solution may be calculated according to the initial volumes of each of its components. Calculations are given per liter of solution, and are then multiplied by the total volume delivered.

For example: a solution containing 400 ml D50, 500 ml 10% aa and 200 ml 20% lipid is calculated as follows:

Dextrose = 400 ml D50 = 400 x 0.5 (% dextrose) = 200 gms
Kcal from dextrose = 200 gms x 3.4 kcal/gm = 680 kcal per liter of solution.

Protein = 500 ml of 10% amino acids = 500 x 0.1 (% a.a.) = 50 gms
Kcal from protein = 50 gms x 4 kcal/gm = 200 kcal per liter of solution.

Lipid = 200 ml of 20% lipid = 200 x 2 kcal/ml = 400 kcal per liter of solution.

Parenteral Nutrition

TOTALS PER LITER
Total kcal per liter = 1280 kcal
Total gms protein/liter = 50 gms
Total gms dextrose/liter = 200 gms

If this solution is given continuously over 24 hours, at a rate of 80 ml/hour, the total volume given will equal 1920 ml. The total amounts for each component must be multiplied by 1.92, giving the following results:

Total Kcal = 1280 kcal x 1.92 = 2,458 kcal
Total protein = 50 gms x 1.92 = 96 gms
Total dextrose = 200 gms x 1.92 = 384 gms

Grams of dextrose in any solution should be within the recommended range for the resident's maximum glucose utilization rate which is calculated using the resident's body weight in grams as follows: 4.3-7.2 gms dextrose/kg body weight/day.

Lipid content should not exceed the maximum recommended rate, which is calculated as follows: 1.5 gms lipid/kg body weight/day.

Protein content should not exceed 25% of total kcal, which can also be calculated as follows: 1.5-2 gm protein/kg body wt/day.

If calcium and phosphorus are added to the solution the sum of the calcium concentration in mEq/L and the phosphate concentration in mMol/L should not exceed 30. This calculation is important to assure a safe administration of the solution; calcium and phosphate ions, if excessive, may form a crystalline precipitate in the solution.

Electrolytes and other additives should be carefully managed according to the specific need of the resident receiving the parenteral nutrition.

Calculation of PPN Solutions

Calculation for components of the PPN solution are similar to that of TPN, however PPN is subject to restrictions that limit the amount of nutrients that can be delivered to the resident. Its primary benefit is to provide enough kcal to prevent catabolism of lean body mass.

Parenteral Nutrition

Since the solution will be administered via a peripheral vein, it must not exceed 900 mOsm/L. Concentrations above this level dramatically increase the risk of phlebitis. Thus lipid becomes the primary source of Kcal for a PPN solution (40-60% of total Kcal). Dextrose is provided in concentrations of 5-10%. The following table provides helpful information for calculating PN solutions:

Component	Kcal/L	mOsm/L	gms/L
10% dextrose	340	504	100
20% dextrose	680	1008	200
5.5% aa	220	575	55
8.5% aa	340	890	85
10% lipids	1100	260	100
20% lipids	2000	260	200
Electrolytes	---	235	---

GLUTEN-FREE DIET

I. **Description**

The Gluten-free diet is a modification of the regular diet. This diet is designed for residents with celiac disease (CD). The diet should be individualized based on the residents needs. Celiac disease is also sometimes referred to as nontropical sprue, celiac sprue, or gluten-sensitive enteropathy. Celiac disease is an autoimmune genetic disorder in which the villi in the duodenum and small intestine are damaged in response to the ingestion of gluten.

Gluten is a storage protein (prolamins) found in all forms of wheat. Strict avoidance of any gluten-containing item is necessary to prevent reoccurrence of symptoms, i.e. bloating, diarrhea, and nausea. Careful review of food items including medications, toothpastes, mouthwashes, lip sticks, communion wafer, as additives, preservatives and stabilizers may contain gluten.

Malabsorption of fat, fat-soluble vitamins, folate, B12, and iron may occur. Supplemental vitamins and minerals should be considered in these cases. In addition, lactose intolerance is common in these cases until the diet is well controlled.

Note: This is not a complete list. Always read food labels. If in doubt, check with the manufacturer.

Food Products	FOODS INCLUDED	Foods in Question	FOODS EXCLUDED
Milk Products	milk, buttermilk, plain yogurt, cheese, cream cheese, cottage cheese	Flavored yogurt, sour cream, frozen yogurt	Malted Milk
Bread, Cereal & Grains	Bread or baked products made from corn, rice arrowroot cornstarch soy, amaranth potato flour, sago, potato starch, tapioca, whole-bean flour, flax, arrowroot, rice bran, buckwheat, millet, teff, cornmeal cornmeal, pea flour, corn tacos, corn tortillas, cassava, garfava, nut flours	Rice crackers, rice cakes, commercial breads	Bread and baked containing wheat, rye, barley, oat bran, bulgur, spelt wheat –based semolina, rye, oats, couscous, triticale, graham flour, semolina wheat flour, durum flour, filler Kamut, imported foods labeled Gluten-free einkorn, seitan, emmer, bromated flour, farina, orzo, phosphate flour, plain flour, white flour, self-rising flour
Cereals	cream of rice, soy cereal, hominy, hominy grits, brown, white and wild rice, cornmeal, quinoa flakes, buckwheat groats, puffed rice, puffed corn	Flour or cereal products	Cereals with wheat, rye, oats, triticale, barley, cereals made with added malt extract and extract and malt flavorings caramel color
Pastas	Macaroni, spaghetti and noodles from rice, quinoa, corn, soy, potato, peas, beans, or other allowed flours.		pastas made from wheat, wheat starch, modified food starch and other ingredients not allowed.

Food Products FOODS INCLUDED Foods in Question FOODS EXCLUDED

Meats & Alternatives

	FOODS INCLUDED	Foods in Question	FOODS EXCLUDED
Meat, fish & Poultry	Fresh, frozen, canned, salted and smoked	Prepared or preserved meats such as ham, luncheon meat, bacon pate, sausages, meat and sandwich spreads, meat product extenders, hot dogs, salami, sausage	Fish canned in vegetable broth containing (HVP) hydrolyzed vegetable & wheat protein or (HPP) hydrolyzed plant protein, turkey basted or injected with HVP/HPP
Eggs	Eggs	Egg substitutes, dried eggs and egg whites	Imitation bacon Imitation seafood
Others	Lentils, chickpeas beans, nuts, tofu, seeds, peas, legumes, sorghum	Baked beans, dry roasted nuts, peanut butter communion wafers	
Fruits	Fresh, frozen canned fruits and fruit juices	Dried fruits, fruit pie filling	
Vegetables	Fresh, frozen or canned veg., yucca	French fried potatoes	Batter dipped vegetables
Soup	homemade broth, gluten-free bouillon, cream soups and stocks made from allowed ingredients.	Canned soups, dried soup mixes, soup base, and bouillon cubes	Soups made with ingredients not allowed. Bouillon containing HPP or HVP
Fats	butter, lard, cream, shortening, margarine, homemade dressing from allowed ingredients	Salad dressing, some mayonnaise	Packaged suet prepared marinades

Food Products	FOODS INCLUDED	Foods in Question	FOODS EXCLUDED
Desserts and Sweets	ice cream, sherbet, ice whipped toppings, egg custard, gelatin, cakes, cookies pastries made with ingredients allowed honey, jam, jelly, sugar	Milk puddings, custard mixes, pudding mixes icing, powdered sugar spreads, candies, chewing gum, lemon lemon curd, marshmallow.	Ice cream with not allowed ingredients. ice cream cones; cakes cookies, pastries made with not allowed ingredients. Licorice, candies with not allowed ingredients.
Snack Foods	Plain popcorn and nuts.	Dry roasted nuts, flavored potato chips, tortilla chips Energy bars	Pizza, unless made with allowed ingredients
Condiments	plain pickles, olives relish, ketchup, mustard, vinegars, pure black pepper, pure spices and herbs, tomato paste, Gluten free soy sauce, modified food starch from tapioca, corn potato	Worcestershire sauce, mixed spices (i.e. curry powder, chili powder)	Soy sauce, mustard pickles, imitation pepper, malt vinegar
Other	sauces and gravies made with allowed ingredients pure cocoa, chocolate chips, MSG, cream of Tartar, coconut, aspartame, baking soda, carob chips and powder, yeast, brewer's yeast, distilled alcoholic beverages, Indian rice grass, Job's tears.	Baking powder, beer	Sauces and gravies made with not allowed ingredients, oat gum.

GLUTEN-FREE SUBSTITUTIONS

Substitution for 1 Tablespoon of Wheat flour.**

½ tablespoon	Cornstarch
½ tablespoon	Potato starch of flour
½ tablespoon	White rice flour
½ tablespoon	Arrowroot starch
2 teaspoon	Quick-cooking tapioca or Tapioca starch
2 tablespoon	Uncooked rice

Substitution of 1 cup wheat flour:

Mix together 2 cups brown rice flour, 2 cups sweet rice flour and 2 cups rice polish. Store in an airtight container and use 7/8 cup of the mixture in place of 1 cup of wheat flour.

**A combination of flours/starches produces a better gluten-free product.

Resource Organizations
Celiac Disease Foundation
13251 Ventura Blvd., Suite 3
Studio City, CA 91604
818-990-2354

1. The American Dietetic Association Manual of Clinical Dietetics, 2002 edition.

2. Miletic ID. Miletic VD. Sasttely-Miller, EA, et al. Identification of gliadin presence in pharmaceutical products. J Pediatr Gastroenterol Nutr. 1994; 19: 27-33

3. Murray, JA. The widening spectrum of celiac disease. Am J Clin Nutr. 1999; 69: 354-365.

4. Case, Shelly-Gluten free diet: a comprehensive resources guide 2004.

FINGER FOOD DIET

Suggested Menu Ideas

PURPOSE   To provide adequate nutrition while promoting independence in eating for individuals with dementia-related diseases, such as Alzheimer's cognitive impairments, or other neuromuscular disorders.

CHARACTERISTICS   A regular diet consistency which can be easily eaten with the fingers and not requiring silverware. It is the policy that finger food meals will be offered to any resident identified as having difficulty efficiently feeding themselves with utensils, possibly leading to risk of poor nutrition.

NUTRITIONAL ADEQUACY   Depending on individual food choices, this diet is adequate in all nutrients.

SERVING SUGGESTIONS   Use of adaptive equipment, such as plate stabilizers, plate guards, "nosey" cups, covered or spouted cups, and cups or mugs with large or double handles may be helpful for some individuals.

Liquids, including soups, cold cereal in milk, or thin, cooked cereal should be served in a mug or with a straw.

Food should be cut in bite-sized pieces, slices, wedges, or made into sandwiches.

Baby carrots, tomato or lettuce wedges, or small pieces or other raw vegetables or fruit are easier to eat.

Whole, fresh fruit may served if the individual can bite off pieces.

Potatoes should be served in pieces that can be picked up easily.

Eggs should be hard cooked (boiled, scrambled or fried).

Dry cereals should be larger pieces served without milk.

FINGER FOOD DIET

Suggested Menu Ideas

Peanut butter should be served on crackers or bread quarters.

Sandwiches, pancakes, waffles, toast, bread, quick breads or cake should be cut into quarters or sliced into sticks.

Foods in sauce or those soft, slippery, crumbly, large or small are hard to handle.

Pasta such as rotini, tortellini, or novelty shapes are recommended because they are thicker and easier to pick up. **Do not overcook or serve in sauce**.

Gravies, sauces, salad dressings or syrup are served in cups so foods can be dipped.

FINGER FOOD DIET

Suggested Menu Ideas

Bread, Cereal & Grains

    Toast (whole wheat, rye, white) brushed with margarine
    Crackers (variety)
    Bread Sticks
    Rolls
    French Toast Strips brushed with margarine
    Waffles/Pancake Strips brushed with margarine
    Plain cold cereals (enriched with vitamins and minerals)
    Cereal/Breakfast Bars (Granola/NutriGrain)
    Muffins
    Pita Bread

Potatoes

    Cubes, slices, wedges
    Tater Tots
    French Fries
    Potato Chips
    Sweet Potatoes (slices or patties)
    Potato Triangles

Fruits

    Sliced, diced, fresh, frozen, canned, or dried

Vegetables

    Salads (may be portioned into pocket pita)
    Baby Carrots
    Green Beans
    Vegetable Strips

Meat/Meat Substitutes

    Hard Boiled Eggs, Deviled Eggs
    Chicken, Beef, Turkey, Pork Strips
    Chicken Nuggets
    Fish Nuggets (Cod, Catfish, Halibut)
    Sausage Link

FINGER FOOD DIET

Suggested Menu Ideas

Dairy Products

Cheese Cubes, Cheese Sticks (variety)
Yogurt/Jello Cubes

Combination Meal

Sandwich sliced into strips or cut in half and placed on each side of plate
Scrambled Egg in Pita Pocket
Egg Sandwich
Casseroles and Stews (may be portioned in a pita pocket)

Desserts

Jello Jigglers
Ice Cream Bars
Ice Cream Sandwiches
Cookies/Cookie Bar (Fortified, if possible)
Cake Squares

Non-finger foods with service/presentation modification

Casseroles served in cereal bowls with soup spoon utensil
Short pasta noodles to replace spaghetti (elbow macaroni, orzo, ziti)
served in cereal bowls
Soup served in mugs

Thickened Liquids

Nectar-like thickened liquids – able to go through straw, glides off a spoon e.g. fruit nectars, shakes, eggnogs.

Honey-like thickened liquids will not go through a straw and will flow slowly off a spoon.

Pudding (spoon thick) – need to be fed with a spoon, of a pudding consistency.

Residents ordered thickened liquids should not be given foods that become liquid at room temperature e.g. gelatin, ice cream, sherbet, water ices.

Follow directions on thickener to achieve desired consistency.

Suggested sites for additional information on thickened liquids and puree foods –

Estimated Caloric Needs – Method I

The following methods for estimating total daily caloric needs may be used as guidelines when assessing the resident's needs. The dietitian must observe for signs of caloric excess or deficiency and make adjustment(s) as needed. In these equations, use the metabolically active weight (MAW) for the obese resident, i.e., 20 percent and 25 percent above ideal body weight (IBW) for women and men respectively. For the resident who is 10 percent or more under ideal body weight, use the ideal body weight. If actual body weight is used in the Harris-Benedict Equation for a resident that is underweight or has experienced significant weight loss, 500 additional calories should be added to the injury and activity factor to promote weight gain. There may be other accepted formulas that are not listed.

Method I This method, based on height, weight, gender and age, can be used for any adult or adolescent.

Step 1. Using the Harris-Benedict Equations, calculate the basal energy expenditure (BEE) in calories.

Male $BEE = 66 + (13.7 \times wt. (kg)) + (5 \times ht. (cm)) - (6.8 \times age)Y$

Female $BEE = 655 + (9.6 \times wt. (kg.)) + (1.8 \times ht. (cm)) - (4.7 \times age)$

Step 2. To calculate the estimated total daily calories (ETDC) needed, multiply the BEE times the activity factor (AF) times the injury factor (IF).
$ETDC = (BEE) \times (AF) \times (IF)$

Estimating Kilocalorie Needs Based on Activity and Injury Factor

Activity Factors (AF):

Bedridden	1.1
Sedentary (no independent movement)	1.2
Active (walks, wheels own wheelchair)	1.3
Seated work, little movement, little leisure activity	1.4 – 1.5
Standing work	1.6 – 1.7
Strenuous work or highly active leisure activity	1.8 – 1.9
30 – 60 minutes strenuous leisure activity 4 – 5 times per week	

Injury (Stress) Factor (IF):

None	1.0
Recent minor surgery	1.1
Recent major surgery	1.2
Wound healing *	1.2 - 1.6
Burns (% total body surface):	
0 – 20	1.00 – 1.50
20 – 40	1.50 – 1.85
40 – 100	1.85 – 2.05
Cancer	1.2 – 1.45
Mild infection/ Stage II pressure sore	1.2
Moderate infection/ Stage III pressure sore	1.3 – 1.4
Severe infection/ Stage IV pressure sore	1.8
Pulmonary disease	1.3
Recent long bone fracture	1.3
Fever (for every degree fever above normal +7% for every 1 degree increase in temperature)	1.7
Multiple trauma with patient on ventilator	1.50 – 1.25
Peritonitis	1.4
Sepsis	1.2 – 1.4
Severe infection/multiple trauma	1.3 – 1.55
Trauma with steroids	1.60 – 1.70

*The dietitian will determine the adjustments required based on the number and severity of decubiti.

Estimated Caloric Needs – Method II

This method of estimating caloric needs addressed only physically healthy persons who are sedentary and moderately active. It is based on body weight, regardless of height, age and gender. It does not allow for injury or stress situations. Physically healthy elderly sedentary residents may require fewer calories for maintenance than used here.

CALORIC LEVELS

Weight Goals	Sedentary	Moderate Activity
Weight Maintenance	30 cal/kg	35 cal/kg
Weight gain	35 cal/kg	40 cal/kg
Weight loss	20-25 cal/kg	30 cal/kg

The above was compiled from:

1. Pocket Resource for Nutrition Assessment. DHCC, 2013.

Estimated Protein Needs

Protein Factors: grams protein /kg body weight
0.8 – 1.0	Average adult (non-stressed)
1.2-1.5	Draining wounds, fracture, or recent major surgery
1.0-1.1	Stage I pressure sore
1.2	Stage II pressure sore
1.3-1.4	Stage III pressure sore
1.5-1.6	Stage IV pressure sore

*Increase fluids & monitor renal function

1.0-1.2	Mildly depleted serum albumin (3.5 – 3.2 mg/dl)
1.2-1.5	Moderately depleted serum albumin (3.2-2.8 mg/dl)
1.5-2.0	Severely depleted serum albumin (<2.8)

Cast Weights:
½ leg	2-4 #
Long leg	4-6 #
Arm	2-3 #
Short arm	1-2 #
Immobilizer	1-2 #

Adjustment in weight for paralysis
Paraplegia 5% - 10% decrease in IBW
Quadriplegia 10% - 15% decrease in IBW

Adjustment of IBW for Amputations
Foot 1.8% \Below knee 6.0%\At knee 9.0%\Above knee 15%\Whole leg 18.5%\
Hand 8%\Forearm & hand 3.1%\Whole arm & Hand 6.5%

Estimated Protein Needs

For the obese resident, i.e., 20 percent and 25 percent above ideal body weight (IBW) for women and men respectively, use the adjusted body weight found elsewhere in the appendix. For the resident who is 10 percent or more below ideal body weight, use the ideal body weight.

Clinical judgment should be utilized when calculating protein needs. The rationale should be documented in the medical record.

Protein Needs

Protein needs may vary depending on a number of factors, including but not limited to;

- Renal status
- Hepatic function
- Presence of metabolic stress (i.e. pressure ulcer or wound, infection, etc.)
- Undernutrition or protein-energy malnutrition (PEM)
- Presence of hepatic (liver) disease

Comprehensive nutrition assessment is needed to determine the appropriate level of protein.

Diseases and Conditions	Protein Needs
Critical illness including burns, sepsis, traumatic brain injury	1.5-2.0 gm/kg/day
GI Issues	
Inflammatory bowel disease	1.0-1.5 gm/kg/day
Short bowel syndrome	1.0-1.2 gm/kg/day
Hepatic disease	
Hepatitis	1.0-1.5 gm/kg/day
Cirrhosis	1.0-1.2 gm/kg/day
Obesity, with hypocaloric feeding:	
BMI>27, normal function of kidneys, liver	1.5-2.0 gm/kg/IBW/day
Class I or II obesity with trauma (ICU)	1.9 gm/kg/IBW/day
Class III obesity with trauma (ICU)	2.5 gm/kg/IBW/day
Pulmonary Disease	1.2-1.5 gm/kg/day
Renal Disease	
Predialysis	0.6-0.8 gm/kg/day
Hemodialysis	1.2-1.3 g/kg, up to 1.5-1.8 gm/kg/day
Peritoneal dialysis	>1.5-2.5 gm/kg/IBW/day
Continuous renal replacement therapy (CRRT	>1.5-2.5 gm/kg/IBW/day
See Renal/Chronic Kidney Disease section of this manual for more detail information	
Stroke	1.0-1.25 gm/kg/day

Miffin - St. Jeor Equation (MSJ) Cheat Sheet

Weight Pounds	kg	MSJ*	Height Feet	Inches	cm	MSJ*	Age Years	MSJ*
85	38.64	386.36	4'9"	57	144.78	904.88	70	350
90	40.91	409.09	4'10'	58	147.32	920.75	72	360
95	43.18	431.82	4'11"	59	149.86	936.63	74	370
100	45.45	454.55	5'	60	152.4	952.50	76	380
105	47.73	477.27	5' 1"	61	154.94	968.38	78	390
110	50.00	500.00	5' 2"	62	157.48	984.25	80	400
115	52.27	522.73	5' 3"	63	160.02	1000.13	82	405
120	54.55	545.45	5' 4"	64	162.56	1016.00	83	410
125	56.82	568.18	5' 5"	65	165.1	1031.88	84	415
130	59.09	590.91	5' 6"	66	167.64	1047.75	85	420
135	61.36	613.64	5' 7"	67	170.18	1063.63	86	425
140	63.64	636.36	5' 8"	68	172.72	1079.50	87	430
145	65.91	659.09	5' 9"	69	175.26	1095.38	88	435
150	68.18	681.82	5' 10"	70	177.8	1111.25	89	440
155	70.45	704.55	5' 11"	71	180.34	1127.13	90	445
160	72.73	727.27	6'	72	182.88	1143.00	91	450
165	75.00	750.00	6' 1"	73	185.42	1158.88	92	455
170	77.27	772.73	6' 2"	74	187.96	1174.75	93	460
175	79.55	795.45	6' 3"	75	190.5	1190.63	94	465
180	81.82	818.18					95	470
185	84.09	840.91					96	475
190	86.36	863.64					97	480
195	88.64	886.36					98	485
200	90.91	909.09					99	490
205	93.18	932.82					100	495
210	95.45	954.55					101	500
215	97.73	977.27					102	510
220	100.00	1000.00					103	515

REE for Males:
* (MSJ weight + MSJ Height - MSJ age) + 5
* **REE for Females:**
(MSJ weight + MSJ Height - MSJ age) - 161
* Always use actual body weight
* Activity factor: 1.20 confined to bed
* Activity factor: 1.30 out of bed / Ambulatory

*Disclaimer – Use discretion when using this formula for resident's that are severely underweight and severely overweight.

Note: According to the American Dietetic Association (ADA) Evidence Analysis Library, if it is not possible to measure RMR, then the Mifflin-St Jeor equation using actual weight is the most accurate for estimating RMR for overweight and obese individuals when BMI is >30.

Male REE = 9.99(wt kg) + 6.25 (ht cm) - (4.92 x age) + 5
Female REE = 9.99(wt kg) + 6.25 (ht cm) – (4.92 x age) - 161

Estimated Fluid Needs

Water requirements is adults range from 1500 to 2000 milliliters (ml) per day with additional needs ranging from 500 to 1500 ml/day if the resident has a fever, fistular draining, wounds, vomiting, diarrhea or excessive perspiration. Also, consider additional fluid is needed when a resident is utilizing an air fluidized bed. Consider water restriction for adults with congestive heart failure, renal failure, cardiac cachexia or hyponatremia. Total daily fluid requirements for residents not needing fluid restriction can be estimated using the following methods:

Method I   This method is based on energy intake in calories regardless of age and weight. This method may be used for residents receiving tube feedings. 1 ml/kcal This calculation underestimates fluid needs in obese patients.

Method II   This method is based on actual body weight in kilograms and age. This method may be used for residents within their ideal body weight.

Age in Years	cc/kg
18-54	30-35 ml/kg actual body weight
55-65	30 ml/kg actual body weight
over 60	25-30 ml/kg actual body weight

Method III   This method may be used for residents who are overweight.

1500 ml for the first 20 kg + 15 ml for every kg over 20 kg

Method IV   This method adjusts for extremes in body weight.

100 ml fluid per kg for the first 10 kg actual body weight
50 ml fluid per kg for the next 10 kg actual body weight
15 ml fluid per kg for the remaining kg actual body weight

*Clinical judgment needs to be utilized when selecting formula to use. The rationale should be documented in the medical record.

This above information was adapted from:

Zeman, F. Clinical Nutrition and Dietetics. 2nd edition, New York: MacMillan Publishing Company, 1991.

Pocket Resource for Nutrition Assessment. DHCC, 2013.

Chidester J.C., Spangler, A.A. "Fluid intake in the institutionalized elderly." J Am Diet Association. 1997.

Estimated Fluid Needs

Clinical assessment for estimating fluid needs: Comparison of intake and output, urine volume and concentration, skin and tongue turgor, dry mucous membranes, body weight, thirst, tearing and salivation, appearance and temperature of skin, edema, temperature, pulse and respiration, blood pressure, neck vein filling, hand vein filing and facial appearance.

Clinical signs of fluid and electrolyte imbalances:
Water deficiency: Loss of skin turgor, dry mucous membranes, increased temperature and pulse, delirium and coma, concentrated urine and thirst. Water excess: Pulmonary and peripheral edema, abdominal and skeletal muscular twitching and cramps, stupor, coma or convulsions.

The above information was adapted from:
Grant, A., DeHoog, S.: <u>Nutritional Assessment and Support.</u> 4th edition, Washington: Northgate Station, 1991.

Serum Osmolality

Osmolality measures the concentration of particles in solution. Osmolality increases with dehydration (loss of water without loss of solutes) and decreases with over hydration.

Greater than normal levels may indicate: Dehydration, Diabetes Insipidus, Hyperglycemia, Hypernatremia, Uremia.

Lower than normal levels may indicate: Hyponatremia, Over hydration, inappropriate ADH secretion.

Normal range is 285-295 mOsm/kg.

Estimated Height (Stature)

Height may be obtained by vertical measurement of the resident standing erect or by measuring the length of a bedfast resident. Either of these figures may be inaccurate due to obesity, shortening with age, and deformities caused by vertebral collapse, arthritis, kyphosis, scoliosis, osteoporosis, contractures, and pulmonary disease, all of which affect trunk length but not limb length. For all adult residents, true stature may be estimated from limb length.

Method I   **Arm Span Measurement**

In adults, a rough estimate (within approximately 10%) of height can be obtained by measuring arm span. The arm span measurement is obtained by fully extending the upper extremities, including the hands, parallel to the floor. The distance between the tip of the middle finger on one hand to the tip of the middle finger on the other hand is measured, providing the arm span, or an estimate height.

If necessary, one arm can be used. With the resident's arm (either) and hand stretched out straight perpendicular to the side, measure the distance from the sternal notch (mid sternum) to the tip of the middle finger of the outstretched hand. Double the figure to obtain the height.

Method II   **Knee Height**

Measure the residents knee height from the bottom of the heel to the top of the knee when the knee is bent at a 90 degree angle and use the following formula to calculate the height.

Male: Height (cm) = 64.19-(0.04 x age)+(2.02 x knee height [cm])

Female: Height (cm) = 84.88-(0.24 x age)+(1.83 x knee height[cm])

The above information was adapted from:

Zeman, Frances J. Clinical Nutrition and Dietetics 2/e. Englewood Cliffs, New Jersey: Macmillan Publishing Company, 1991.

Pocket Resource for Nutrition Assessment. DHCC, 2013.

Estimating height from ulna length

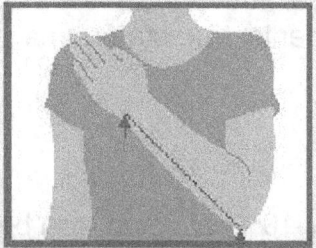

Measure between the point of the elbow and the midpoint of the prominent bone of the wrist (left side if possible). Height in meters is determined from the following chart, based on the ulna length as measured in cm.

Men(<65years)	1.94	1.93	1.91	1.89	1.87	1.85	1.84	1.82	1.80	1.78	1.76	1.75	1.73	1.71
Men(>65years)	1.87	1.86	1.84	1.82	1.81	1.79	1.78	1.76	1.75	1.73	1.71	1.70	1.68	1.67
Ulna length(cm)	32.0	31.5	31.0	30.5	30.0	29.5	29.0	28.5	28.0	27.5	27.0	26.5	26.0	25.5
Women(<65years)	1.84	1.83	1.81	1.80	1.79	1.77	1.76	1.75	1.73	1.72	1.70	1.69	1.68	1.66
Women(>65years)	1.84	1.83	1.81	1.79	1.78	1.76	1.75	1.73	1.71	1.70	1.68	1.66	1.65	1.63

Men(<65years)	1.69	1.67	1.66	1.64	1.62	1.60	1.58	1.57	1.55	1.53	1.51	1.49	1.48	1.46
Men(>65years)	1.65	1.63	1.62	1.60	1.59	1.57	1.56	1.54	1.52	1.51	1.49	1.48	1.46	1.45
Ulna length(cm)	25.0	24.5	24.0	23.5	23.0	22.5	22.0	21.5	21.0	20.5	20.0	19.5	19.0	18.5
Women(<65years)	1.65	1.63	1.62	1.61	1.59	1.58	1.56	1.55	1.54	1.52	1.51	1.50	1.48	1.47
Women(>65years)	1.61	1.60	1.58	1.56	1.55	1.53	1.52	1.50	1.48	1.47	1.45	1.44	1.42	1.40

Nutrition Assessment Guidelines: When Adjustments Are Required

Ideal Body Weight (IBW)
Men: IBW=106 pounds (lb) for first 5 feet + 6 lb for each inch over 5 feet
Women: IBW=100 lb for first 5 feet + 5 lb for each inch over 5 feet
For the individual shorter than 5 feet, subtract 2 lb for each inch under 5 feet

IBW frame size adjustment
Add or subtract 10% IBW
Large Frame: IBW + (IBW x 0.10)
Small Frame: IBW – (IBW x 0.10)

Adjustment for patients with disabilities
Paraplegia: Subtract 5%-10% from IBW
Quadriplegia: Subtract 10%-15% from IBW

Consultant Dietitians in Health Care Facilities, CD-HCF Pocket Resource for Nutrition Assessment, 2005 Revision.

Adjustment For Patients With Amputations

Use the percentage of total body weight contributed by individual body parts:

Body Part	Percentage
Trunk without extremities	50.0%
Entire leg (and foot)	16.0%
Below the knee	6.0%
Foot	1.5%
Entire arm (and hand)	50.0%
Forearm	2.3%
Hand	1.0%

Obesity is usually defined as 125% or more of ideal (IBW) or a Body Mass Index (BMI)>30. Since body fat is not nearly as metabolically active as other tissue using actual body weight to calculate caloric needs will result in a figure that is too high. Alternatively, using Ideal Body Weight (IBW) to calculate caloric needs will result in a figure that is too low because it will not take into account the additional lean body mass to support the excess weight or extra calories needed to move it.

The following equation may be used to obtain the metabolically active weight (MAW) for estimating total daily calorie and protein requirements. This calculation is not used to calculate fluid needs. Actual body weight should be used to calculate fluid needs.

$$MAW = [(Actual\ Body\ Weight) - IBW) \times 0.25] + IBW$$

The above information was adapted from:

Mahan, L. Kathleen and Arlin, Marian. <u>Krause's Food, Nutrition & Diet Therapy,</u> ~~8th edition.~~ Philadelphia: W. B. Saunders Company, 1992.

Energy Requirements for Adults

Energy prediction equations
For resting energy expenditure (REE) or resting metabolic rate (RMR), where weight (W) in kilograms (KG), height (H) in centimeters and age (A) in years.

Ireton-Jones
Legend:
- B=Diagnosis of burn (present=1, absent=0)
- O=Obesity, body mass index (BMI>27kg/m2 (present=1, absent=0)
- S=Sex (male=1, female=0)
- T=Diagnosis of trauma (present=1, absent=0)

Spontaneously Breathing: 629-11(A)+25(W)-609(O)
Ventilator-Dependent (original, 1992): 1925-10(A)+5(W)+281(S)+292(T)+851(B)
Ventilator-Dependent (revised, 2002): 1784-11(A)+5(W)+244(S)+239(T)+804(B)

Owen
Note: Indirect calorimetry is the preferred method for determining RMR in critically ill patients. If it is necessary to use predictive equations, according to ADA evidence-based practice guidelines, the **Ireton-Jones** (1992) is one of the equations cited as having the best prediction accuracy. **Harris-Benedict and Mifflin-St Jeor** are not recommended for critically ill patients.

Men: 879+(10.2xW)
Women: 795+(7.18xW)

Total energy requirements

Total energy requirements (TEE)=REE x(activity factor) x (injury factor) +/- 500 calories (for desired weight loss or weight gain, if applicable) + fever factor

Activity factors (AF)
Comatose 1.1
Confined to bed: 1.2
Confined to chair: 1.25
Out of bed: 1.3

Injury factors (IF):
Surgery
Minor: 1.0-1.2
Major: 1.1-1.3
Skeletal trauma: 1.6-1.8
Head Trauma: 1.6-1.8
Pressure ulcers
Stage I: 1.0-1.1
Stage II: 1.2
Stage III: 1.3-1.4
Stage IV: 1.5-1.6
Infection
Mild: 1.0-1.1
Moderate: 1.2-1.4
Severe: 1.4-1.8
Burns (% body surface area)(BSA)
<20% BSA: 1.2-1.5
20%-40% BSA: 1.5-1.8
>40% BSA: 1.8-2.0
Fever factor

Fahrenheit scale: add 7% of REE for every 1 degree over normal
Centigrade scale: add 13% of REE for every 1 degree over normal

References and Recommended Readings

Breen HB, Ireton-Jones CS. Predicting energy needs in obese patients. *Nutr. Clin Pract.* 2004; 19:284-289.

Campbell CG, Zander E, Thorland W. Predicted vs measured energy expenditure in critically ill underweight patients. *Nutr Clin Pract.* 2005; 20: 276-280.

Frankenfield D, Roth-Yousey L, Compher C. Comparison of predictive equations for resting metabolic rate in healthy non-obese adults and obese adults: a systematic review. *J Am Diet Association.* 2005; 105: 775-789.

Ireton-Jones CS, Jones JD. Improved equations for predicting energy expenditure in patients: The Ireton –Jones equations. *Nutr Clin Pract.*2002; 17:29-31.

Ireton-Jones CS, Turner WW Jr, Leipa GU, Baxter CR. Equations for estimation of energy expenditures in patients with burns with special reference to ventilator status. *J Burn Care Rehabil.* 1992:13: 330-333.

Monoamine oxidase (MAO) inhibitors are antidepressants which can cause dangerous reactions such as hypertensive crisis when taken with foods containing tyramine, dopamine, alcohol and caffeine. It is recommended that the diet continue for four weeks following discontinuation of the drug.

MAO Inhibitors
Examples
Brand (Generic Name) Marplan (isocarboxazid)
Nardil (Phenelzine)   Eldepryl (selegiline)
Parnate (Tranylcypromine)

Foods and Beverages to Avoid
Aged cheeses:

Cheddar	Processed	
Camembert	Gruyere	Boursault
Emmenthaler	Gouda	Parmesan
Swiss	Natural brick	Romano
Stilton	Mozzarella	Provolone
	Bleu	Imitation cheese

Beer   Vermouth
Ale   Ginseng
Wine   Alcohol free and reduced
                  Alcohol beer and wine products

Salted, dried cod and herring
Pickled herring
Meat extracts and bouillons
Summer sausage
Any unfresh meat, stored or aged beef, aged game
Beef or Chicken livers
Fermented (hard) sausage
Bologna
Pepperoni
Salami
Italian broad beans
Excessive amounts of chocolate and caffeine (coffee, tea, and cola)
Overripe fruit, banana peel
Marmite yeast, yeast extracts, Brewers yeast
Liquid and powdered protein supplements
Hydrolyzed protein extracts used as a base for sauces, soups or gravies
Fermented bean curd and soya bean paste, miso (Use soy sauce with caution.)
Fava Beans
Avocados

Foods and drinks low in tyramine may be consumed with reason, but never in excess. They include caffeine containing drinks, chocolate, soy sauce, cottage cheese, cream cheese, yogurt and sour cream.

This information was compiled from:

Manual of Clinical Dietetics, Yale-New Haven Hospital. New Haven: Department of Food and Nutritional Services, 1990.

Physician's Desk Reference 53rd edition. Montvale: Medical Economics Data, 1999.

Pronsky, Z.M., Food Medication Interactions. Birchrunville, PA. 14th Edition, 2006

Drug Facts and Comparisons. Facts and Comparisons, 2000. Applied therapeutics: The Clinical Use of Drugs, Applied Therapeutics, 1995. The American Psychiatric Press Textbook of Psychopharmacology. American Psychiatric Press, Inc., 1998.

Fiber Content of Common Foods

Food Item	Serving Size	Total Fiber per serving (g)	Soluble Fiber per serving (g)	Insoluble Fiber per serving(g)
Cereals				
All Bran	1/3 cup	8.6	1.4	7.2
Cheerios	1 ¼ cup	2.5	1.2	1.3
Corn flakes	1 cup	0.5	0.1	0.4
Cream of wheat, Regular (uncooked)	2 ½ tbsp	1.1	0.4	0.7
Fiber one	½ cup	11.9	0.8	11.1
40% Bran flakes	2/3 cup	4.3	0.4	3.9
Grapenuts	¼ cup	2.8	0.8	2.0
Grits, corn, quick (uncooked)	3 tbsp	0.6	0.1	0.5
Oat bran (cooked)	¾ cup	4.0	2.2	1.8
Oat bran flakes	½ cup	2.1	0.8	0.3
Oatmeal (uncooked)	1/3 cup	2.7	1.4	1.3
Product 19	1 cup	1.2	0.3	0.9
Puffed rice	1 cup	0.2	0.1	0.1
Puffed wheat	1 cup	1.0	0.5	0.5
Raisin bran	¾ cup	5.3	0.9	4.4
Rice Krispies	1 cup	0.3	0.1	0.2
Shredded wheat	2/3 cup	3.5	0.5	3.0
Shredded wheat & bran	2/3 cup	2.5	0.6	1.9
Special K	1 cup	0.9	0.2	0.7
Total, whole wheat	1 cup	2.6	0.6	2.0
Wheaties	2/3 cup	2.3	0.7	1.6
Grains				
Cornmeal	2 ½ tbsp	0.4	0.1	0.3
Macaroni, white (cooked)	½ cup	0.7	0.4	0.3
Macaroni, whole wheat (cooked)	½ cup	2.1	0.4	1.7
Noodles, egg (cooked)	½ cup	1.4	0.4	1.0
Popcorn, popped (cooked)	3 cups	2.0	0.1	1.9
Rice, white (cooked)	1/3 cup	0.5	trace	0.5
Spaghetti, white (cooked)	½ cup	0.9	0.4	0.5
Spaghetti, whole wheat (cooked)	½ cup	2.7	0.6	2.1
Wheat bran	½ cup	12.3	1.0	11.3
Wheat germ	3 tbsp	3.9	0.7	3.2

Fiber Content of Common Foods

Food Item	Serving Size	Total Fiber per serving (g)	Soluble Fiber per serving (g)	Insoluble Fiber per serving (g)
Bread and Crackers				
Bagel, plain	½	0.7	0.3	0.4
Biscuit, baked	1	0.5	0.3	0.2
Bread	1 slice	0.7	0.3	0.4
Bran muffin	1 muffin	1.8	0.2	1.6
Cornbread	2 in	1.4	0.3	1.1
Cracked, wheat	1 slice	1.9	0.3	1.6
French	1 slice	0.9	0.3	0.6
Mixed grain	1 slice	1.9	0.3	1.6
Pita, white	½ pocket	0.5	0.2	0.3
Pumpernickel	1 slice	2.7	1.2	1.5
Raisin	1 slice	1.8	0.8	1.0
Rye	1	1.8	0.8	1.0
White	1 slice	0.6	0.3	0.3
Whole wheat	1 slice	1.5	0.3	1.2
Bun, hamburger	½	0.7	0.2	0.5
Crackers, matzo	1	1.0	0.5	0.5
Saltine	6	0.5	0.3	0.2
Saltine, wheat	5	0.5	0.2	0.3
Snack, whole wheat	4	2.0	0.3	1.7
Wheat	5	0.6	0.2	0.4
English muffin	½	0.8	0.2	0.6
Pretzels, hard	¾ oz	0.8	0.2	0.6
Rolls, brown-and-serve	1 roll	0.8	0.3	0.5
Taco shell	2	1.4	0.2	1.2
Tortilla, corn	1	1.4	0.2	1.2
Tortilla, flour	1	0.7	0.3	0.4
Waffle, toasted	1	0.7	0.3	0.4

Fiber Content of Common Foods

Food Item	Serving Size	Total Fiber per serving (g)	Soluble Fiber per serving (g)	Insoluble Fiber per serving (g)
Fruits				
Apple, red, fresh with skin	1 small	2.8	1.0	1.8
Applesauce, canned Unsweetened	½ cup	2.0	0.7	1.3
Apricots, canned, drained	4 halves	1.2	0.5	0.7
Apricots, dried	7 halves	2.0	1.1	0.9
Apricots fresh, with skin	4	3.5	1.8	1.7
Avocado, fresh, flesh only	1/8	1.2	0.5	0.7
Banana, fresh	½ small	1.1	0.3	0.8
Blueberries, fresh	¾ cup	1.4	0.3	1.1
Cherries	½ cup	1.8	0.9	0.9
Dates, dried	2 ½ medium	0.9	0.3	0.6
Figs, dried	1 ½	2.3	1.1	1.2
Fruit cocktail, (canned)	½ cup	2.0	0.7	1.3
Grapefruit, fresh	½ medium	1.6	1.1	1.2
Grapes, red, fresh With skin	15 small	0.4	0.2	0.2
Kiwifruit, fresh, flesh only	1 large	1.7	0.7	1.0
Melons, cantaloupe	1 cup cubed	1.1	0.3	0.8
Melons, honeydew	1 cup cubed	0.9	0.3	0.6
Melons, watermelon	1 ¼ cup cubed	0.6	0.4	0.2
Nectarine, fresh	1 small	1.8	0.8	1.0
Orange, fresh	1 small	2.9	1.8	1.1
Peaches	½ cup	3.7	0.7	3.0
Pears	½ cup	3.7	0.7	3.0
Pineapple, canned	1/3 cup	1.4	0.2	1.2
Plum, red, fresh	2 medium	2.4	1.1	1.3
Prunes	3 medium	1.7	1.0	0.7
Raisins, dried	2 tbsp	0.4	0.2	0.2
Raspberries, fresh	1 cup	3.3	0.9	0.2
Strawberries, fresh	1 ¼ cup	2.8	1.1	1.7

Fiber Content of Common Foods

Food Item	Serving Size	Total Fiber per serving (g)	Soluble Fiber per serving (g)	Insoluble Fiber per serving(g)
Vegetables				
Asparagus, (cooked)	½ cup	1.8	1.7	1.1
Bean sprouts, fresh	1 cup	1.6	0.6	1.0
Beets, flesh only(cooked)	½ cup	1.8	0.8	1.0
Broccoli, (cooked)	½ cup	2.4	1.2	1.2
Brussels sprouts(cooked)	½ cup	3.8	2.0	1.8
Cabbage, fresh	1 cup	1.5	0.6	0.9
Cabbage, red (cooked)	½ cup	2.6	1.1	1.5
Carrots, (canned)	½ cup	1.5	0.7	0.8
Carrots, fresh	7 ½ in long	2.3	1.1	1.2
Carrots, sliced (cooked)	½ cup	2.0	1.1	0.9
Cauliflower, (cooked)	½ cup	1.0	0.4	0.6
Celery, fresh	1 cup chopped	1.7	0.7	1.0
Corn, whole kernel (canned)	½ cup	1.6	0.2	1.4
Cucumber, fresh	1 cup	0.5	0.2	0.3
Green beans (cooked)	½ cup	2.0	0.5	1.5
Kale, chopped, frozen	½ cup	2.5	0.7	1.8
Lettuce, iceberg	1 cup	0.5	0.1	0.4
Mushrooms, fresh	1 cup pieces	0.8	0.1	0.7
Okra, frozen (cooked)	½ cup	4.1	1.0	3.1
Olives, (canned)	10 small	1.0	0.1	0.9
Onion, fresh, (chopped)	½ cup	1.7	0.9	0.8
Peas, green (canned)	½ cup	3.2	0.4	2.8
Peas, green, frozen (cooked)	½ cup	4.3	1.3	3.0
Pepper, green, fresh	1 cup chopped	1.7	0.7	1.0
Potato, sweet (canned)	1/3 cup	0.8	0.3	0.5
Potato, white, flesh only (cooked)	½ cup	1.5	0.3	1.2
Pumpkin, canned	½ cup	3.5	0.6	2.9
Snow peas, fresh(cooked)	½ cup	1.4	0.6	0.8
Spinach (cooked)	½ cup	1.6	0.5	1.1
Squash, yellow, crookneck, frozen	½ cup	1.3	0.5	0.4

Fiber Content of Common Foods

Food Item	Serving Size	Total Fiber per serving (g)	Soluble Fiber per serving (g)	Insoluble Fiber per serving(g)
Vegetables				
Tomato (canned)	½ cup	1.3	0.5	0.8
Tomato, fresh	1 medium	1.0	0.1	0.9
Tomato, sauce	1/3 cup	1.1	0.5	0.6
Turnip (cooked)	½ cup	4.8	1.7	3.1
V-8 juice	½ cup	0.7	0.2	0.5
Zucchini, sliced (cooked)	½ cup	1.2	0.5	0.7
Legumes				
Black beans (cooked)	½ cup	6.1	2.4	3.7
Black-eyed peas (canned)	½ cup	4.7	0.5	4.2
Butter beans, dried (cooked)	½ cup	6.9	2.7	4.2
Chick peas (canned)	½ cup	4.3	1.3	3.0
Kidney beans, dark, red dried, cooked	½ cup	6.9	2.8	4.1
Lentils, dried (cooked)	½ cup	5.2	0.6	4.6
Lima beans (canned)	½ cup	4.3	1.1	3.2
Navy beans, dried, (cooked)	½ cup	6.5	2.2	4.3
Pinto beans (canned)	½ cup	6.1	1.4	4.7
Split peas, dried (cooked)	½ cup	3.1	1.1	2.0
White beans, Great Northern (canned)	½ cup	7.2	2.2	5.0
Nuts and Seeds				
Almonds	6 whole	0.6	0.1	0.5
Brazil nuts	1 tbsp	0.5	0.1	0.4
Coconut, dried	1 ½ tbsp	1.5	0.1	1.4
Coconut, fresh	2 tbsp	1.1	0.1	1.0
Hazelnuts, (filberts)	1 tbsp	0.5	0.2	0.3
Peanut butter, smooth	1 tbsp	1.0	0.3	0.7
Peanuts, roasted	10 large	0.6	0.2	0.4
Sesame seeds	1 tbsp	0.8	0.2	0.6
Sunflower seeds	1 tbsp	0.5	0.2	0.3
Walnuts	2 whole	0.3	0.1	0.2

RECIPES FOR FIBER SUPPLEMENTS

BRAN-PRUNE JUICE SUPPLEMENT

Yield: 32 oz   Serving size: 1-4 oz/day

9 oz bran buds
23 oz prune juice
1 cup unsweetened applesauce

Combine all ingredients in a large blender. Blenderize until well mixed. Cover, label with date and time processed. Discard after 72 hours.
Total dietary fiber per ounce: 2.23 gm.

OATMEAL WITH BRAN

Yield: 14 cups   Serving size: ½ cup
21 oz oatmeal
9 oz bran buds

Cook oatmeal according to directions. When cooked, add bran. Stir, and serve immediately.
Total dietary fiber per serving: 4.06 gm.

PRUNE WHIP

Yield: 16 oz   Serving size: 1 oz

1 cup unsweetened applesauce

1 cup unprocessed bran, all bran or bran buds
½ cup prune juice
2 tablespoons honey

Combine all ingredients and blend until smooth. Cover and label product with date and time processed. Store in refrigerator. Discard after 72 hours.
Total dietary fiber per ounce: 2.2 gm.

CAFFEINE CONTENT OF FOODS AND BEVERAGES

Item	Caffeine/mg Range	Item	Caffeine/mg Range
Coffee (5 oz cup) Brewed Nuts and Seeds		**Chocolate Products**	
Drip	110-150	Cocoa hot (5 oz)	2-15
Percolated	40-70	Cocoa dry (1 oz)	6
Decaffeinated	2-5	Chocolate milk (8 oz)	8
Coffee (5 oz cup) Instant		Milk chocolate (1 oz)	1-15
Freeze, dried	40-108	Dark chocolate, semi-sweet (1 oz)	5-35
Decaffeinated	2-3		
Tea (bags or loose) (5 oz)		Bakers chocolate (1 oz)	25
1 minute brew	9-33	Chocolate-flavored syrup (2 tbsp)	5
3 minute brew	20-46		
5 minute brew	20-50	Chocolate malted, milk powder (3 heaping tbsp)	8
Tea Products			
Instant (5 oz cup)	12-29	Chocolate chips, semi-sweet (2 oz)	12-15
Iced tea (12 oz cup)	22-36	**Soft Drinks, Diet (12 oz)**	
Soft Drinks, Regular (12 oz)		Tab	46
Mello Yellow, Mountain Dew, Kick	52-55	Diet Cola, Dr. Pepper	36-59
		Soft Drinks, Diet (12 oz)	
Soft Drinks, Regular (12 oz)		Tab	46
Mello Yellow, Mountain Dew, Kick	52-55	Diet Cola, Dr. Pepper	36-59
Cola, Dr. Pepper, Barqs, Root Beer	35-46	Sugar-free Big Red	38
Pepsi, RC Cola, Big Red, Aspen	18-38	Diet Mr. Pibb	40
Mr. Pibb	40	Canada Dry Diet Cola, Fresca	1-4

CAFFEINE CONTENT OF FOODS AND BEVERAGES

Item Range	Caffeine/mg	Item Range	Caffeine/mg
Club soda, Seltzer, Sparkling water, Caffeine-free cola, Ginger ale, Sprite, Slice Fresca, 7-Up, Root beer, Orange, Grape, Strawberry, Power Aide, tonic water	0	Caffeine-free Diet Cola Diet Sprite, Diet Slice, Diet Orange, Diet Root Beer, Diet 7-Up	0
Jolt	72	Jolt	72 mg
Orange Slice	40-48	Diet Orange slice	40-48 mg
Coke Zero	45		
Pepsi Max	43		

Scoop Sizes

Number	Approximate Liquid Volume
6	2/3 cup (5 fluid ounces)
8	½ cup (4 fluid ounces)
10	3/8 cup (3 ¼ fluid ounces)
12	1/3 cup (2 2/3 fluid ounces)
16	¼ cup (2 fluid ounces)
20	3 1/5 tablespoons (1 3/5 fluid ounces)
24	2 2/3 tablespoons (1 1/3 fluid ounces)
30	2 1/5 tablespoons (1 fluid ounce)
40	1 3/5 tablespoons (0.8 fluid ounce)
60	1 tablespoon (0.5 fluid ounce)

Scoops, also called dippers, are used to measure volume not weight. Originally used to measure and serve ice cream, each scoop's number indicates the number of serving found in a quart (32 fluid ounces) of ice cream. For example, using a number eight scoop, eight half-cup servings (4 fluid ounces each) would be obtained from a quart of ice cream. Two number 8 scoops of ice cream equals one cup (8 fluid ounces) but weighs only 4.7 ounces.

Milligram and MilliEquivalent Conversions

Formula for converting milligrams (mg) to milliEquivalents (mEq):

$$\frac{\text{milligrams}}{\text{atomic weight}} \times \text{valence} = \text{milliEquivalents}$$

Example: $\frac{1000 \text{ mg Na}}{23} \times 1 = 43 \text{ mEq}$

Formula to use when converting milliEquivalents (mEq) to milligrams (mg):

$$\frac{\text{milliEquivalents} \times \text{atomic weight}}{\text{valence}} = \text{milligrams}$$

Example: $\frac{60 \text{ mEq K} \times 39.1}{1} = 2346 \text{ milligrams}$

Mineral	Atomic Weight	Valence
Zinc (Zn+)	65.4	2
Sodium (Na+1)	23.0	1
Potassium (K+)	39.1	1
Calcium (Ca+1)	40.1	2
Chlorine (C1-)	35.5	1
Phosphorus (P-)	31.0	2
Magnesium (Mg+)	24.3	2
Sulfur (S-1)	32.1	2

<u>Salt and Sodium Conversions</u>
To convert milligrams of sodium (Na+) to milligrams of salt (NaCl):
    sodium milligram ÷ .40 = salt milligrams

To convert milligrams of salt (NaCl) to milligrams of sodium (Na):
    Salt milligrams x .40 = sodium milligrams

1 teaspoon salt (5gm) = 2300 mg Na
1 salt packet (5/8 gm) = 288 mg

Measures and Metric Conversions

Liquid measure – volume equivalent

1 teaspoon	=	1/3 tablespoon	=	5 ml
1 tablespoon	=	3 teaspoons	=	15 ml
2 tablespoons	=	1 fluid ounce	=	30 ml
8 tablespoons	=	½ cup	=	120 ml
16 tablespoons	=	1 cup (8 fluid ounces)	=	½ pint, 240 ml
2 cups	=	1 pint (16 fluid ounces)	=	.4732 liters
2 pints	=	1 quart (32 fluid ounces)	=	.9462 liters
1.06 quarts	=	34 fluid ounces	=	1000 ml
4 quarts	=	1 gallon	=	3785 ml

Dry measure-volume equivalent

1 quart	=	2 pints	=	1.101 liters

Dry measure and quarts are about 1/6 larger than liquid measure pints and quarts.

Linear measure

1 inch	=	2.54 centimeters (rounded to 2.5)

Weights

Avoirdupois		Metric
1 ounce	=	28.32 grams (rounded to 30)
1 pound (16 ozs)	=	453.6 grams (rounded to 454)
1 pound (16 ozs)	=	.45 kilogram
2.2 pounds	=	1 kilogram

Conversions

kilograms x 2.2	=	pounds (lb)
pounds x 0.4	=	kilograms (kg)
inches x 2.5	=	centimeters (cm)
centimeters 2.5	=	inches (in)
grams x 1000	=	milligrams (mg)
liter x 1000	=	millilters (ml)
liter x 100	=	centiliter (cl)
liter x 10	=	deciliter (dl)

Note: "Ounce" may mean 1/16 of a pound or 1/16 of a pint; however, the former is weight measure and the latter is volume measure. Except for water (or other substances with the same density as water), a fluid ounce and a weight ounce are not equivalent and should not be used interchangeably.

Abbreviations

The following official and unofficial abbreviations are used frequently in residents' medical records. This list should be modified according to the facility's policies for approved abbreviations.

a.	before	ml	milliliter
a.c.	before food or meals	N.P.O.	nothing by mouth
ad lib	as desired		nothing may pass orally
A.D.L.	activities of daily living	OOB	out of bed
A.S.C.V.D.	arteriosclerotic cardiovascular disease	.T.	occupational therapy
A.S.H.D.	arteriosclerotic heart disease	OTC	over the counter
b.m.	bowel movement	oz	ounce
p.r.n.	whenever necessary, or	p.c.	after meals
B.M.R.	basal metabolism rate	p.o.	postoperative or by mouth at patient request
B.P.	blood pressure	P.T.	physical therapy
B.S.	bowel sounds	q	every
B.U.N.	blood urea nitrogen	q.h.	every hour
c	with	R.B.C.	red blood count
Ca	calcium	R/O	rule out
CA	cancer	R.O.M.	range of motion
C.B.C.	complete blood count	Rx	prescription, treatment
C.H.F.	congestive heart failure	S	without
CHO	carbohydrate	S.O.B.	shortness of breath
C.N.S.	central nervous system	S.S.	soap suds
C.O.	complains of	stat	immediately
C.V.A.	cerebrovascular accident	tbsp	tablespoon
D/C	discontinue	t.i.d.	three times a day
DX	diagnosis	T.P.R.	temperature, pulse and respiration
E.E.G.	electroencephalogram		
E.K.G.	electrocardiogram	tsp	teaspoon
E.N.T.	ear, nose, throat	U.R.I.	upper respiratory infection
F.B.S.	fasting blood sugar		
gd	good	UTI	urinary tract infection
gm	gram	wt.	weight
gr	grain		
gtt	drop		
hgb	hemoglobin		
hct	hematocrit		
h.s.	bedtime		
lb	pound		
lt	liter		
mEq	milliEquivalent		

Official "Do Not Use" List

Do Not Use	Potential Problem	Use Instead
U (unit)	Mistaken for "O" (zero), the Number "4" (four) or "cc"	Write "unit"
IU (International Unit)	Mistaken for IV (intravenous) or the number 10 (ten)	Write "International Unit"
Q.D., QD, q.d., qd (daily)	Mistaken for each other	Write "daily"
Q.O.E., QOD, q.o.d, qod (every other day)	Period after the Q mistaken for "I" and the "O" mistaken for "I"	Write "every other day"
Trailing zero (X.0 mg)* Lack of leading zero (.X mg)	Decimal point is missed	Write X mg Write 0.X mg
MS	Can mean morphine sulfate or Magnesium sulfate	Write "morphine sulfate" Write "magnesium sulfate"
MSO4 and MgSO4	Confused for one another	

1 Applies to all orders and all medication-related documentation that is handwritten (including free-text computer entry) or on pre-printed forms.

*Exception: A "trailing zero" may be used only where required to demonstrate the level of precision of the value being reported, such as for laboratory results, imaging studies that report size of lesions, or catheter/tube sizes. It may not be used in medication orders or other medication-related documentation.

Additional Abbreviations, Acronyms and Symbols
(For possible future inclusion in the Official "Do Not Use" List)

Do Not Use	Potential Problem	Use Instead
>(greater than)	Misinterpreted as the number	Write "greater than"
<(less than)	"7" (seven) or the letter "L"	Write "less than"
Abbreviations for drug names	Confused for one another Misinterpreted due to similar Abbreviations for Multiple drugs	Write drug Names in full
Apothecary units	Unfamiliar to many Practitioners Confused with metric units	Use metric units
@	Mistaken for the number "2" (two)	Write "at"
cc	Mistaken for U (units) when poorly written	Write "ml" or "milliliters"
ug	Mistaken for mg (milligrams) resulting in one thousand-fold overdose	Write "mcg" or

RECIPES FOR PUREE BREAD

Pureed Bread

Bread	2 ½ loaves
Broth	1 gallon
Margarine	¼ lb

Season to taste

In steam table, pan break bread slices into small pieces
Pour broth/melted margarine mixture over bread
Lightly mix bread and liquid together
Bake uncovered at 325 degrees F. until browned – approximately 20 minutes

Hold at 145 degrees F. or above

Yield: 40 servings - #12 scoop

Variations:

Add ground pepper, pureed onion and celery
Choose broth flavor depending on meat served

Example: seafood broth, beef, pork or poultry broth
Season with sage, poultry seasoning, garlic powder or Old Bay seasoning to compliment meal

Recipe – Pureed Bread, Warm

Yield: 25   Size of Serving: 1/3 cup

AMOUNT	INGREDIENT	PREPARATION STEP
8 1/3 cup	Japanese Bread Crumbs	1. Combine margarine, milk, water and chicken base in sauce pan. Simmer over medium heat just until margarine has melted. Remove from heat. Add bread crumbs, mix thoroughly until all bread crumbs are moistened.
½ gal	Milk, 2% low fat	
1 3/8 cup	Water #1	
½ cup	Margarine, hard stick	
1 3/8 tbsp	Chicken base	

2. Let bread mixture stand for 5 minutes to transfer to a greased 2" deep hotel pan. **Note** Length of pan required will depend on number of servings prepared. Cover pan with plastic wrap.

3. Cook in steamer for 20 minutes or until internal temperature reaches 165 degrees for 15 seconds.

4. Portion with a #12 scoop for service.

Recipe – Pureed Bread, Cold

Yield: 25	Size of Serving: 1/3 cup

AMOUNT	INGREDIENT	PREPARATION STEP
8 1/3 cup	Japanese Bread Crumbs	1. Combine margarine, milk, water and chicken base in sauce pan. Simmer over medium heat just until margarine has melted. Remove from heat. Add bread crumbs, mix thoroughly until all bread crumbs are moistened.
½ gal	Milk, 2% low fat	
1 3/8 cup	Water #1	
½ cup	Margarine, hard stick	
1 3/8 tbsp	Chicken base	
1 pint	Water #2	

2. Let bread mixture stand for 5 minutes transfer to a greased 2" deep hotel pan. **Note** Length of pan required will depend on number of servings prepared. Cover pan with plastic wrap.

3. Cook in steamer for 20 minutes or until internal temperature reaches 165 degrees for 15 seconds.

4. Cool the bread in refrigerator until it reaches an internal temperature of 40 degrees or below.

5. Prior to service, add water to the cooled bread mixture stirring until the mixture is a smooth mashed potato consistency.

6. Portion with a #12 scoop for service.

Recipe – Pureed Bread, Cinnamon

Yield: 25	Size of Serving: 1/3 cup	Cost per serving: $
Cooking Time:	Temperature:	Method: (None)

AMOUNT   **INGREDIENT**   **PREPARATION STEP**

AMOUNT	INGREDIENT
8 1/3 cup	Japanese Bread Crumbs
½ gal	Milk, 2% low fat
1 3/8 cup	Water #1
½ cup	Margarine, hard stick
½ cup	Sugar, Granulated
1/3 Tsp	Cinnamon, Ground

1. Combine margarine, milk, water in sauce pan. Simmer over medium heat just until margarine has melted. Remove from heat. Add bread crumbs, sugar and cinnamon mix thoroughly until all bread crumbs are moistened.

2. Let bread mixture stand for 5 minutes. Transfer mixture to a greased 2" deep hotel pan. **Note** Length of pan required will depend on number of servings prepared. Cover pan with plastic wrap.

3. Cook in steamer for 20 minutes or until internal temperature reaches 165 degrees for 15 seconds.

4. Portion with a #12 scoop for service.

Pureed Bread

Portion Size: #16 Scoop
Number of Servings: 24

Ingredients	Amount	Unit
Wheat Bread	24	Slices
Apple Juice	12	Ounces
Hot water	12	Ounces

Procedure	CCP	Monitor	Corrective Action
1. Place slices of Wheat bread in food processor.			
2. Add hot water and blend for approximately 30 seconds.			
3. Add fruit juice and continue to blend. You may add flavoring or spices at this time also.			
4. Hot serve. Heat in Steamer.	CCP	Monitor	Corrective Action Temp of 165° for 15 sec.
5. Transfer to steam table at time of service. Serve with #16 scoop.	CCP	Measure temp.	If temperature falls to less than 140° F. reheat food to 165° F. one time only.
6. Cold Serve: Transfer product to shallow pan and cool from 140° to 70° in 2 hours and from 70° to 40° in 4 hours. Portion and serve during service #16 scoop.	CCP	Monitor temp.	Chill by approved method to 40°

(NOTES)

Optional variations:
Cinnamon ¼ tsp. to every 12 slices bread
Vanilla flavoring ½ tsp. to every 12 slices of bread
Orange or cranberry juice may be substituted for apple juice for variety.

(DIABETIC EXCHANGES)

#16 scoop = 1 CHO/Bread

FRENCH TOAST SOUFFLE

May be used for a puree diet and/or to add calories

16 slices white bread without crust
1   8 ounces block of cream cheese
8 pasteurized eggs or liquid equivalent
1 ½ cups milk
2/3 cup Half and Half
½ cup maple syrup (light syrup is okay)
1 teaspoon vanilla
Cinnamon to taste
Serve with powdered sugar and maple syrup

1. Spray a 13 x 9 baking dish with cooking spray/Pam
2. Rip bread into quarters and place in baking dish
3. Beat cream cheese at medium speed until smooth
4. Add eggs, one at a time, mixing after each addition
5. Add milk, creamer, maple syrup, vanilla, and cinnamon
6. Pour mixture over bread, cover, and refrigerate overnight
7. Preheat oven to 375 degrees
8. Let bread mixture stand at room temperature for 15 minutes
9. Tent aluminum foil over dish and bake for 40 minutes
10. Remove foil and bake another 10 minutes or until golden brown
11. Sprinkle with powdered sugar and serve with maple syrup

SUPER SHAKE

120 ml provides approximately 200 calories and 6 grams protein.

SUPER SHAKE RECIPE

Number of 120 ml servings	9
Carnation Instant Breakfast	2 packs
Whole milk	1 cup (8 ounces)
Evaporated Milk	1 can (13 ounces)
Ice Cream	1 ½ - 8 ounce scoop
Corn Syrup	½ cup

Types of Mental Health Issues

What is schizophrenia?

Schizophrenia is a major mental disorder that affects many people. About one in every one hundred people (1%) develops the disorder at some time in his or her life. It occurs in every country, every culture, every racial group and at every income level.

Schizophrenia causes symptoms that can interfere with many aspects of people's lives, especially their work and social life. Some symptoms make it difficult to know what's real and what's not real. These symptoms have been described as being similar to "dreaming when you are wide awake." Other symptoms can cause problems with motivation, concentration, and experiencing enjoyment.

It is important to know that there are many reasons to be optimistic about the future:

- There is effective treatment for schizophrenia.
- People with schizophrenia can learn to manage their illness.
- People with schizophrenia can lead productive lives.

What is bipolar disorder?

Bipolar disorder is a major mental illness that affects many people. It is sometimes called "manic depression." About one person in every one hundred people (1%) develops the disorder at some time in his or her life. It occurs in every country,
every culture, every racial group and at every income
level.

Bipolar disorder causes symptoms that can interfere with many aspects of people's lives. Some of the
symptoms cause severe mood swings, from the highest of highs (mania) to the lowest of the lows (depression.) Some of the other symptoms of
bipolar disorder can make it difficult to know what's real and what's not real (psychotic symptoms).

It is important to know that there are many reasons to be optimistic about the future:

- There is effective treatment for bipolar disorder.
- People with bipolar disorder can learn to manage their illness.

What is depression?

Depression is one of the most common psychiatric disorders. 15 to 20 people out of every 100 have a period of serious depression at some time in their lives. It occurs in every country, every culture, every racial group and at every income level.

Depression causes people to have extremely low moods, when they feel very sad or "blue." It can also cause problems in appetite, sleeping and energy level. For some people, depression can seriously interfere with their work and social life.

It is important to know that there are many reasons to be optimistic about the future:

- There is effective treatment for depression
- People with depression can learn to manage their own illness
- People with depression can lead productive lives.

Introduction

Using alcohol, such as drinking a beer, a glass of wine, or a mixed drink, is common in modern society. Similarly, using certain types of street drugs is also common, such as marijuana, cocaine, amphetamines ("speed"), and hallucinogens (such as LSD and "ecstasy"). Although using these types of substances can make people feel good, they can also cause problems and make it more difficult for people to manage their psychiatric illness. This module focuses on the effects of drug and alcohol use on mental illness and other parts of life, and offers strategies for reducing these effects.

Commonly Used Substances and Their Effects

It is helpful to understand what people commonly experience when they use alcohol and drugs. The following table lists both the positive and negative effects of alcohol and drugs.

Developing a Sober Lifestyle

When people decide to develop a sober lifestyle, it takes planning and practice. Sometimes there can be setbacks along the way, such as urges to use substances or relapses in substance use. Developing your own personal plan for a sober lifestyle is an important part of managing your mental illness and achieving your personal recovery goals. There are three important steps to achieving sobriety:

- Remember your reasons for not using substances.
- Develop a plan to prevent going back to using substances in "high risk" situations.
- Identify new ways of getting your needs met.

Tips for accomplishing each of these steps are provided below:

Identifying Personal Reasons For Not Using Substances

Whenever someone decides to cut down or stop using substances, it is important for them to identify their personal reasons for wanting a sober lifestyle, and to regularly remind themselves of these reasons. In what ways could sobriety help you achieve your personal recovery goals? Consider possible reasons such as:
- Better ability to manage mental illness (fewer relapses)

What is stress?

"Stress" is a term people often use to describe a feeling of pressure, strain, or tension. People often say that they are "under stress" or feel "stressed out" when they are dealing with challenging situations or events.

Everyone encounters stressful situations. Sometimes the stress comes from something positive (like a new job, new apartment, or new relationship) and sometimes from something negative (like being bored, having an argument with someone, or being the victim of crime).

Stress is the feeling of pressure, strain or tension that comes from dealing with challenging situations.

Question: What is it like when you experience stress?

Disclaimer Statement

All information and content contained in this book are provided solely for general information and reference purposes. Smith Show Publishing LLC Limited makes no statement, representation, warranty or guarantee as to the accuracy, reliability or timeliness of the information and content contained in this Book.

Neither Smith Show Publishing Limited or the author of this book nor any of its related company accepts any responsibility or liability for any direct or indirect loss or damage (whether in tort, contract or otherwise) which may be suffered or occasioned by any person howsoever arising due to any inaccuracy, omission, misrepresentation or error in respect of any information and content provided by this book (including any third-party books.

Cooking Notes

Cooking Notes

Cooking Notes

Cooking Notes

Cooking Notes

Cooking Notes

Cooking Notes

Cooking Notes

Cooking Notes

Cooking Notes

Cooking Notes

Cooking Notes

Cooking Notes

www.ingramcontent.com/pod-product-compliance
Lightning Source LLC
Chambersburg PA
CBHW081721100526
44591CB00016B/2452